Club Drugs and Novel Psychoactive Substances

Over the last decade many hundreds of new psychoactive drugs have emerged onto illicit markets. This flood of new drugs has led to clinicians being unsure of the rapidly emerging changing evidence base and uncertain of the best approaches to assessment and clinical management. This book provides a concise, accessible summary of these emerging drugs. By categorizing the hundreds of new drugs by their predominant psychoactive effect – sedative, stimulant and hallucinogenic – the book helps clinicians to manage a drug they are unfamiliar with by using their experience of other drugs with similar psychoactive properties. Written for clinicians from across the frontline, from A&E staff to drug treatment professionals, the authors draw on numerous clinical examples from their own clinical experiences to illustrate aspects of assessment and management. Club drugs and novel psychoactive substances will continue to challenge clinicians and this handbook provides readers with an invaluable introduction to this complex area.

Owen Bowden-Jones is Consultant in Addiction Psychiatry and Founder of the CNWL Club Drug Clinic, London, and Honorary Professor at University College London. He is Chair of the Advisory Council on the Misuse of Drugs and National Clinical Adviser to the Alcohol, Drugs and Tobacco division at Public Health England.

Dima Abdulrahim is Programme Manager and Principal Researcher for the NEPTUNE Project for the Club Drug Clinic, Central and North West London NHS Foundation Trust. She has been working in the drug treatment field for over 30 years.

Club Drugs and Novel Psychoactive Substances

The Clinician's Handbook

Owen Bowden-Jones
Central North West London NHS Foundation Trust

Dima Abdulrahim
Central North West London NHS Foundation Trust

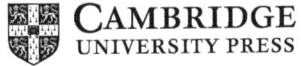
CAMBRIDGE
UNIVERSITY PRESS

CAMBRIDGE
UNIVERSITY PRESS

University Printing House, Cambridge CB2 8BS, United Kingdom

One Liberty Plaza, 20th Floor, New York, NY 10006, USA

477 Williamstown Road, Port Melbourne, VIC 3207, Australia

314-321, 3rd Floor, Plot 3, Splendor Forum, Jasola District Centre, New Delhi - 110025, India

103 Penang Road, #05-06/07, Visioncrest Commercial, Singapore 238467

Cambridge University Press is part of the University of Cambridge.

It furthers the University's mission by disseminating knowledge in the pursuit of education, learning and research at the highest international levels of excellence.

www.cambridge.org
Information on this title: www.cambridge.org/9781911623090
DOI: 10.1017/9781911623106

© Cambridge University Press 2020

First published 2020

A catalogue record for this publication is available from the British Library

Library of Congress Cataloging in Publication data
Names: Bowden-Jones, Owen, author. | Abdulrahim, Dima, author.
Title: Club drugs and novel psychoactive substances : a clinical handbook / Owen Bowden-Jones,
Central North West London NHS Foundation Trust, Dima Abdulrahim, Central North West
London NHS Foundation Trust.
Description: Cambridge, United Kingdom ; New York, NY : Cambridge University Press, 2020. |
Includes bibliographical references and index.
Identifiers: LCCN 2020026282 (print) | LCCN 2020026283 (ebook) | ISBN 9781911623090
(paperback) | ISBN 9781911623106 (ebook)
Subjects: LCSH: Designer drugs. | Psychotropic drugs. | Drugs of abuse.
Classification: LCC RM316 .B69 2020 (print) | LCC RM316 (ebook) | DDC 615.7/88–dc23
LC record available at https://lccn.loc.gov/2020026282
LC ebook record available at https://lccn.loc.gov/2020026283

ISBN 978-1-911-62309-0 Paperback

Contents

Acknowledgements

Thanks to Sarah Finley for her assistance with the critical care sections.

Introduction

1.1 Why Read This Book?

Over the last decade, the UK, Europe and beyond have seen a dramatic change in the patterns of illicit drug use, particularly in adolescents and those in their twenties for whom heroin and crack cocaine have steadily lost popularity (Figure 1.1). While younger drug users continue to use established drugs such as powder cocaine and MDMA, some are attracted to a range of newly emerging drugs, including so-called club drugs and new psychoactive substances.

Worldwide, the last decade has seen an unprecedented increase in the number of substances and combinations available to users through illegal drug markets.[1] [2]

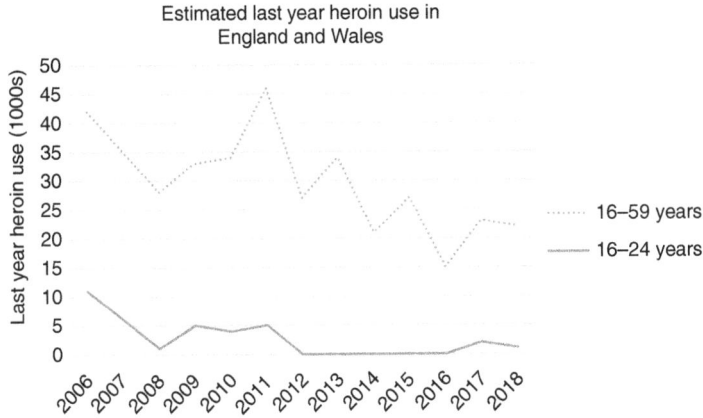

Figure 1.1 Estimated number of people who used heroin in the last year: 16–24 year olds vs 16–59 year olds. Crime Survey England and Wales.

Many of these emerging drugs have poorly understood harms, and as a result clinicians are often unsure of the best method(s) of clinical management. The rapid emergence of numerous new psychoactive drugs in particular is a challenge, as the research evidence to inform clinical management lags far behind the need for clinical care. This lack of evidence-based guidance leaves clinicians without sufficient support in clinical decision making and is a significant problem across the clinical front line.

Club Drugs and Novel Psychoactive Substances: The Clinician's Handbook is intended to provide clinicians from a range of disciplines with a concise summary of this complex emerging field. Offering advice on clinical assessment and management supported by clinical examples, this book is intended to help busy clinicians quickly gain expert knowledge and clinical competence in common clinical presentations.

As this book will clearly demonstrate, the illicit drug market is currently evolving rapidly. Established illicit drugs, newly emerging illicit drugs and non-prescribed and diverted prescription medications are all being made available, increasingly through online or social media platforms. This situation will continue to challenge clinicians for the foreseeable future.

1.2 Aim and Structure

This volume aims to provide clinical information to frontline clinicians in an accessible, clear and rigorous manner in order to improve knowledge and clinical competence in a rapidly emerging area. The book is structured to enable ease of use, with chapters divided by psychoactive effect. Anonymised case studies from the authors' clinical experiences are provided to illustrate key clinical issues. References are provided for those who seek further detail.

There is extensive clinical guidance available for opiate drugs such as heroin, but surprisingly little on the more commonly used 'club' drugs. This book will tackle this knowledge gap by addressing emerging novel psychoactive substances (NPS) and club drugs, including cocaine, MDMA and ketamine. In this way, the reader will gain an overview of emerging drug harms, ranging from established club drugs to the latest NPS.

What Are Club Drugs and NPS and Why Are They Important?

2.1 What Are Club Drugs and NPS?

Drug use patterns over the last decade have been characterised by the emergence of a huge number of new illicit drugs. These drugs include so-called 'club drugs' and 'novel' or 'new' psychoactive substances (NPS), although neither term fully captures the range and complexity of the substances or the ways that they are used. There can be significant overlap between different drugs, but Figure 2.1 demonstrates how they can be considered as established drugs, established club drugs and NPS.

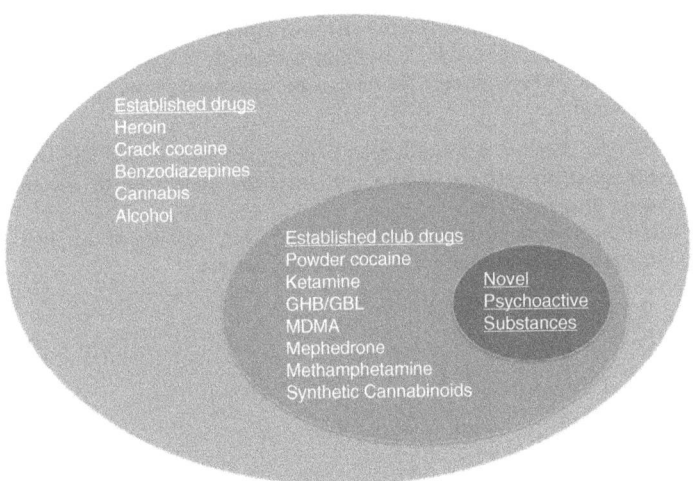

Established drugs
Heroin
Crack cocaine
Benzodiazepines
Cannabis
Alcohol

Established club drugs
Powder cocaine
Ketamine
GHB/GBL
MDMA
Mephedrone
Methamphetamine
Synthetic Cannabinoids

Novel Psychoactive Substances

Figure 2.1 Categorising drugs: Established drugs of misuse, established club drugs and novel psychoactive substances.

2.2 Club Drugs

The term 'club drug' is described by the National Institute of Drug Abuse as a group of psychoactive substances typically used by teenagers and young people at bars, nightclubs, concerts and parties.[3] The term is used to refer to a diverse group of substances with different actions. They include substances that are well established in drug markets, such as MDMA and cocaine, novel psychoactive substances, such as synthetic cathinones and synthetic cannabinoid receptor agonists (SCRAs), and other drugs, such as methamphetamine, well established elsewhere in the world but which has only appeared on the UK and European recreational drug scene in recent years. Confusingly, club drugs are not exclusively used in club or party settings and may be used alone, particularly if problematic use develops.

2.3 Novel Psychoactive Substances

New or novel psychoactive substances can be considered a sub-group of club drugs as they are also largely used in dance venues, house parties and to facilitate sexual behaviours. They are characterised by being rapidly emerging substances often designed specifically to avoid legal control, something that has caused significant concern to policy makers and clinicians and that appears to have recently distorted drug markets in an unprecedented manner. The United Nations Office for Drugs and Crime (UNODC) defines these substances as follows:

> 'Substances of abuse, either in a pure form or a preparation, that are not controlled by the 1961 Single Convention on Narcotic Drugs or the 1971 Convention on Psychotropic Substances, but which may pose a public health threat'.

The term 'new' does not necessarily refer to new inventions, several NPS were first synthesized decades ago, but to substances that have recently become available on drug markets.[4]

Taken together, these two groups include the vast majority of the emerging illicit drugs misused in the UK, Europe and beyond.

Chapter 3

A Brief History of NPS Production and Distribution

3.1 Overview

New psychoactive substances began to cause concern around 2008 when a number of new and diverse drugs were detected on global drug markets. The initial aim of these new drugs appeared to be to mimic the psychoactive effect of established illicit drugs such as MDMA and cocaine, while avoiding legal sanctions to enable their sale by high street vendors.

Over the following six years the European drug market saw an alarming escalation in the number, potency, availability and harms of these drugs. In 2014, 101 drugs were detected on the European drug market for the first time. Policy and enforcement experts were understandably worried about these changes, particularly as the emerging drugs appeared to be aimed at younger users, often with specific branding, packaging and marketing (Figure 3.1).

Clinicians in particular experienced significant challenges. For many years clinicians had only needed expertise in a handful of established, 'traditional' drugs. As new drugs emerged, there was an absence of high-quality research to guide clinicians on the most appropriate assessment and management. For many new drugs all that was available in the research literature were a few case studies. This absence of clinical guidance was highlighted in a number of surveys of clinicians' confidence and competence in managing emerging new drugs.[5]

As of December 2019, more than 950 substances have been reported to the UNODC Early Warning Advisory (EWA) on NPS.[4] In Europe, by the end of 2018 more than 730 new psychoactive substances were monitored, 55 of which were detected for the first time in 2018. These substances make up a broad range of drugs, such as synthetic cannabinoids, stimulants, opioids and benzodiazepines.[6]

As mentioned earlier, the apparent goal of these emerging drugs was to mimic the effects of existing established illicit drugs while at the same time evading legal control. Synthetic substances were specifically manufactured to avoid legal control, often by altering chemical structures to ensure the substance evaded regulatory frameworks. Even small structural modifications to existing illicit drugs could place the modified substance outside legal control. In most cases, however, the structural changes were not significant enough to change the basic pharmacology or the desired psychoactive effects.

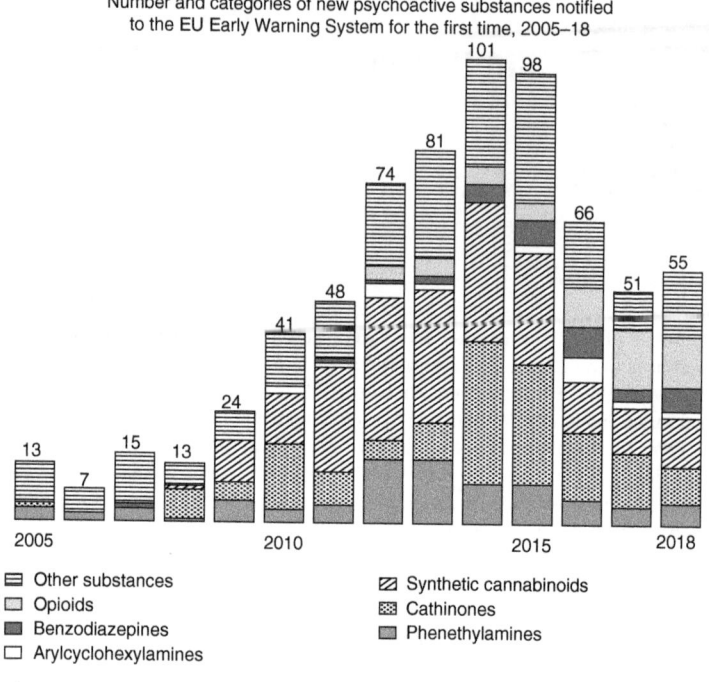

Figure 3.1 Number and categories of NPS in Europe.[6]

The legal status of many of these drugs allowed them to be marketed in a different manner to established illicit drugs. High street vendors began to openly sell NPS with recognised psychoactive effects and known physical and psychiatric harms. Attractive branding was developed to appeal particularly to younger people, and these drugs became widely described as 'legal highs' (Figure 3.2).

In response to the large number of legal psychoactive drugs made available on drug markets, the UK and many other countries initially resorted to using existing mechanisms to place emerging drugs under legal control. These mechanisms often worked by carefully assessing the potential risk of an individual drug (or group of similar drugs) before setting out legislation to bring the specific drug under control. However, the sheer number of new drugs overwhelmed these regulatory mechanisms and drug producers

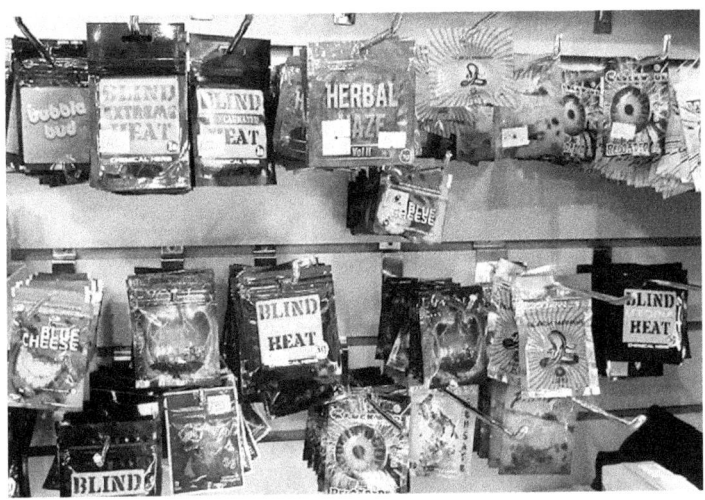

Figure 3.2 'Legal highs' available for sale in high street shops.

engaged in a cat-and-mouse game of bringing new drugs to market as soon as an existing one was controlled. As a result, many countries began to explore new legislative options.

Some countries have issued new legislation regarding NPS, in the form of blanket bans (all NPS), generic bans (groups of NPS with similar chemical structures) and analogue-based controls (individual drugs with structural and psychoactive effects similar to existing controlled drugs). This may have created a more restrictive legal environment, with a subsequent reduction in high street sales and a stabilisation in the number of NPS detected in Europe in recent years.

In the UK, the 2016 Psychoactive Substance Act (PSA) established a blanket ban on all existing and future NPS based on their potential for psychoactive effect. A recent review of the impact of the PSA reported the elimination of high street vendors with some displacement to other markets, including online sellers.

Many NPS have been specifically developed to mimic the effects of more established drugs such as cannabis, cocaine, heroin, LSD, MDMA and methamphetamine, but at lower cost and higher purity. NPS, how-ever, are not the same as the drugs they mimic and have differing chemical properties which determine onset, duration of psychoactive effect, potency and toxicity. Although NPS are sometimes marketed as an alternative or 'legal' version of established drugs, some NPS are also substituted and mis-sold as the original drug in an attempt to increase profits.

3.2 Successive Generations of NPS

As NPS have appeared over the years, new formulations of these substances have become available, with a second, third or even fourth 'generation' being developed. In many cases, these later-generation drugs are more potent than earlier forms and may be associated with greater harms. A good example is SCRAs: initially developed in an attempt to mimic the effects of natural cannabis through agonism of the CB1 receptor, successive generations of SCRAs have become increasingly potent and toxic.

3.3 Change and Continuity

Proliferation of NPS appears rapid and dynamic. Some substances have been detected across many countries and territories and have become established in local drug markets over a number of years, suggesting that substances may persist in the market over time.[6] Other NPS are detected only briefly or in limited geographical areas and then rapidly disappear – for example, bromo-dragonfly, which was reportedly considered too potent by most users.[7]

3.4 Case Study: A Dynamic Market – the Rise and Fall of Mephedrone in the UK

The rapid increase in the use of mephedrone in 2009 in the UK was reported by a number of studies. It was suggested that this increase was associated with the poor quality of cocaine and MDMA at the time. Its popularity was also enhanced by its relative low cost and easy availability due to its 'legal' status before 2010, as well as its effects somewhat similar to MDMA.[8] [9] [10]

Mephedrone use rapidly increased and by 2011/12 was the fourth most popular illicit drug in the UK.[11] It continued to be popular for a number of years, but its use seems to have declined more recently. Treatment data from England show an 88% reduction in people presenting to treatment with problematic use of mephedrone from 2015/16 to 2017/18, with the greatest falls among the youngest groups.[12] Deaths in England and Wales where mephedrone was implicated also decreased from 44 in 2014 to 2 in 2018.[13] There was also a reduction in the number of seizures of mephedrone, which fell by 67%, from 202 in 2016/17 to 66 in 2017/18. This continues the longer-term decline since 2012/13, when there were 3,850 seizures.[14]

3.5 Evolving Drug Markets: New versus Traditional

Three overarching themes have been identified to describe drug markets.[15] These themes apply to both established drugs such as heroin and cocaine and emerging drugs such as club drugs and NPS.

- The increasing organisational and technical complexity, interconnectedness and specialisation of groups involved in making and selling drugs for the drug markets.
- Globalisation and technology as tools to accelerate the rate of change in the drug market, particularly the internet.
- Drug market-related activities are concentrated in a number of established and emerging geographical locations.

The European Monitoring Centre for Drugs and Drug Addiction (EMCDDA) publication on drug markets in Europe has reported that innovation in synthetic drug production and changes in cannabis cultivation have resulted in greater opportunities for drugs to be produced nearer to consumer markets in the EU. Nevertheless, some specific geographical locations or 'hotspots' remain particularly important for drug production or trafficking. Some of these areas are long established, while new zones are also emerging.

3.6 The Role of the Internet

In addition to the traditional physical illicit drugs markets, the internet (both the 'darknet' and the 'clearnet') is now occupying a growing role in the sale of drugs. In Europe, drug sales volumes on darknet markets are currently modest when compared with current estimates of the annual retail value of the overall EU drug market. However, they are significant and have the potential to grow.

An EMCDDA publication reported that the UK together with Germany and the Netherlands were the most important countries with respect to EU-based darknet drug supply in the period between 2015 and 2017. Stimulant drugs represented the majority of all online European drug sales, particularly MDMA and cocaine. It seems that the vast majority of sales originating from the EU between 2011 and 2015 were from these three countries: Germany, with an estimated EUR 26.6 million in total sales; the UK, with just over EUR 20.3 million in total sales; and the Netherlands, with just over EUR 17.9 million in total sales. It has been suggested that darknet markets will most commonly used for mid- or low-volume market sales or sales directly to consumers. Large-volume sales (wholesale) are relatively uncommon.[16]

There is also some evidence that NPS, as well as traditional drugs, are sometimes acquired through social media. The most commonly used technology to acquire drugs is that of mobile phones. Phone-based drug-delivery services, sometime known as 'ring and bring' drug phone lines or 'dial-a-drug' are increasingly common, and an EMCDDA (2018) report described how the European market for cocaine is undergoing a process of 'Uberisation', where more sellers provide 'fast delivery anywhere at any time'.[17]

Chapter

Classification Framework for Club Drugs and NPS

Hundreds of new substances have emerged in the last decade. For most clinicians, it is not possible to develop expertise in each and every existing NPS, or those likely to emerge in the future.

In order to overcome this problem, it is useful to be able to classify these emerging drugs into different groups of substances and allow for linkage to existing treatment protocols. Drugs can be classified using a variety of approaches – for example, chemical structure or pharmacological action; however, for clinicians perhaps the most useful method of categorisation is according to primary psychoactive effect.

The three main psychoactive effects produced by illicit (and legal) drugs are **depressant, stimulant** and **hallucinogenic.** The advantage of using these effects to categorise club drugs and NPS is that clinicians will already be aware

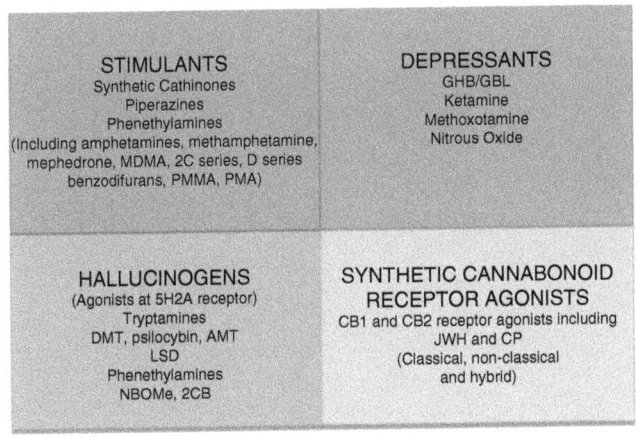

Figure 4.1 Classification of drugs according to psychoactive effect.

of established illicit drugs in each of these groups – for example depressants such as heroin, stimulants such as cocaine and hallucinogens such as LSD. Clear evidence-based protocols exist for the identification and management of established drugs in each of the three psychoactive categories.

Unknown emerging drugs can be similarly categorised using these three psychoactive groups. Capitalising on the clinician's existing knowledge of established drugs, a careful assessment of clinical signs and symptoms will assist in deciding which broad psychoactive category a new drug falls under. This should help clinicians place an unfamiliar drug into a familiar category. In this way a framework for responding to emerging drugs can be quickly developed, even if it only supports initial clinical management.

Although most emerging club drugs and NPS will be predominately depressant, stimulant or hallucinogenic, some will display complex psychoactive effects from more than one psychoactive category. An example is SCRAs, sometimes referred to as synthetic cannabinoids, which do not easily fit into any one psychoactive group due to their chemical, pharmacological and psychoactive diversity. To assist clinicians in the management of SCRAs, we have classified them as a fourth, separate category (See Figure 4.1).

5

The Clinical Challenge of Club Drugs and NPS

5.1 Initial Assessment of the Health Harms of Club Drugs and NPS

The clinical assessment framework for club drugs and NPS is largely the same as for all psychoactive drugs. This book focuses on adverse health effects, but it is important to remember that although outside the scope of this book, assessment of adverse effects should include consideration of social morbidities such as loss of employment and stable housing.

Box 5.1 outlines the areas which should form the assessment of any person using any psychoactive substance.

Box 5.1 Drug Misuse Assessment Should Include (Amended from Drug Misuse and Dependence: UK Guidelines on Clinical Management)[18]

1. Identifying, and responding, to any emergency or acute problem.
2. Confirming the patient is taking psychoactive substances (based on history, examination and drug testing, and through accessing any relevant additional information from clinical records).
3. Identifying degree of problem use or dependence, including:
   - types of psychoactive drugs used (including prescribed and over-the-counter medicines)
   - quantity and frequency of use
   - pattern of use
   - routes of administration (including any injecting)
   - sources of drugs obtained
   - co-ingestion of other drugs/alcohol/prescribed medication
   - environmental conditions in which the drug is consumed
   - evidence for harmful use or dependence (including any experience of withdrawal syndromes).
4. Types of alcohol consumed, quantity and frequency of use, pattern of use, and whether there is evidence of hazardous drinking (above

---

recommended levels for low-risk drinking), or of harmful or dependent use (including experience of alcohol withdrawal syndrome).

5. Identifying current or previous physical problems, including: current or previous physical complications of drug and alcohol use, such as infection with blood-borne viruses or continuing related risk behaviours, liver disease, abscesses, overdoses, enduring severe physical disabilities and sexual health problems.

6. Identifying current or previous psychological or psychiatric problems, such as personality problems and disorders, self-harm, history of abuse or trauma, depression, anxiety and severe psychiatric comorbidity.

7. Identifying current or previous social problems, including: problems in personal relationships (including with partners) and of social integration, including domestic violence and abuse; family, housing and living arrangements; education; employment; and benefits and financial problems.

8. Childcare issues, including parenting, pregnancy and child protection. Risks related to pregnancy. For drug-misusing parents or other adults with dependent children, obtaining information on the child(ren) and any drug-related risks to which they may be exposed. Use child or adult safeguarding procedures as indicated by risk assessment.

9. Criminal involvement, offending and other legal issues, including arrests, fines, outstanding charges and warrants, probation, imprisonment, violent offences and criminal activity, and involvement with workers in the criminal justice system.

10. Assessing the family history for substance use and dependence and relevant medical, psychiatric or psycho-social factors.

11. Determining the patient's understanding of treatment options and motivation for change; exploring and identifying strengths, including personal, family, social and other strengths and positive networks that the service user can use to achieve their treatment and recovery goals.

12. Assessing risk behaviours, including those associated with injecting.

13. With young people, assessing competency to consent to treatment (if required) and involving those with parental responsibility as appropriate.

5.2 Categorising Adverse Health Harms of Club Drugs and NPS

5.2.1 Acute and Chronic Health Harms of Club Drugs and NPS

The adverse effects of all drugs can be considered in terms of acute adverse effects and adverse effects resulting from repeated use. The World Health Organisation's

International Classification of diseases associates different substances with the following primary clinical syndromes: 1) single episode of harmful substance use, 2) harmful pattern of substance use and 3) substance dependence.[19]

5.2.2 Acute Harms

Acute harms occur during or immediately after consumption of the drug. Examples include direct toxicity (overdose) and accidents while intoxicated.

5.2.3 Harms from Repeated Use

These adverse effects are associated with frequent and prolonged use of a particular drug or drugs. Examples include physiological dependence and psychiatric disorders, such as depression.

The World Health Organisation [19] has described two sub-groups of chronic harms – 'harmful use' and 'dependent use' – and these are determined by the severity of the harm experienced by the drug user. They are defined as follows.

Harmful use is a pattern of drug use that has caused damage to a person's physical or mental health or has resulted in behaviour leading to harm to the health of others. The pattern of drug use is evident over a period of at least 12 months if substance use is episodic or at least 1 month if use is continuous (i.e., daily or almost daily).

Harm to health of the individual occurs due to one or more of the following:

1. behaviour related to intoxication,
2. direct or secondary toxic effects on body organs and systems, or
3. a harmful route of administration.

Harm to health of others includes any form of physical harm, including trauma, or mental disorder that is directly attributable to behaviour related to drug intoxication on the part of the person to whom the diagnosis of harmful pattern of use of drug applies.

Dependence is a disorder of regulation of drug use arising from repeated or continuous use of the drug. The characteristic feature is a strong internal drive to use the drug, which is manifested by impaired ability to control use, increasing priority given to use over other activities and persistence of use despite harm or negative consequences. These experiences are often accompanied by a subjective sensation of urge or craving to use the drug. Physiological features of dependence may also be present, including tolerance to the effects of the drug, withdrawal symptoms following cessation or reduction in use of the drug, or repeated use of the drug or pharmacologically similar substances to prevent or alleviate withdrawal symptoms. The features of dependence are usually evident over a period of at least 12 months but the diagnosis may be made if drug use is continuous (daily or almost daily) for at least 1 month.[19]

5.3 Five Specific Clinical Challenges in Assessing Adverse Health Effects of Club Drugs and NPS

Although it is essential to undertake the comprehensive assessment for drugs outlined in Box 1, people who have consumed club drugs and NPS present particular challenges for the clinician.

5.3.1 Unknown Substance at Time of Clinical Presentation

Club drugs and NPS present a unique challenge for clinicians. In most cases, both clinician and patient will be unaware what drug or drugs have been consumed and therefore what potential harms should be anticipated. The chemical content of all illicit drugs is of course unpredictable; however, the large and varied number of emerging drugs and their often similar appearance (e.g. a white powder or branded tablet) reduces the likelihood that a user will know what they have consumed.

5.3.2 Lack of Available Testing

Despite attempts to develop rapid oral fluid or urine testing for emerging club drugs and NPS to be used in clinical settings, the obvious challenge is the large number of available substances and the constant production of new substances. At present there are no available tests, usable at the clinical front line, which can detect all NPS, and it is unlikely that these will be developed in the foreseeable future. In this situation, clinicians will instead need to rely on careful clinical assessment to better understand the harm an individual patient may be experiencing.

5.3.3 Insufficient Evidence on Potential Harms

The research literature on harms for most NPS is very limited, and at best may only consist of case studies or case series; this leaves clinicians with little information on which to base clinical care. The assumption that a new NPS will cause similar harm to another drug in the same class is a good starting point, but successive generation of NPS tend to increase in potency with greater associated harms.

5.3.4 Insufficient Evidence on Clinical Interventions

The evidence for effective clinical interventions for NPS is even less developed than the understanding of the harms different NPS may cause. In most cases, clinicians will have to consider evidence-based interventions and guidance developed for established drugs when managing NPS harms. This will be discussed in detail throughout the volume.

5.3.5 Poly-Drug Use

Many club drug and NPS users will co-ingest multiple substances, including alcohol, during an episode of use. Combining multiple psychoactive substances will potentially influence clinical presentation. Co-ingestion of sedative and stimulant substances can be particularly challenging for the clinician, as presentation may include aspects of both toxidromes simultaneously.

5.4 Overview of the Management of Club Drug and NPS Harms

As discussed, the clinical management of drug harms is complicated by the uncertainty of what has been consumed; the lack of rapid, reliable technology to test for specific NPS; and, in most cases, the lack of pharmaceutical antidotes. The next sections describe clinical approaches to both acute and chronic adverse health effects for different drug groups.

5.4.1 Acute Adverse Health Effects

UK Readers: For up-to-date guidance on the management of acute toxicity, it is recommended that information be sought from the National Poisons Information Service (NPIS), specifically the NPIS 24-hour telephone service and the poisons information database TOXBASE®.

International Readers: Clinicians reading this document should consult their local or national Poisons Information Services and their national and/or local guidelines and protocols on treatment.

5.4.2 Psycho-Social Interventions

Evidence-based psycho-social interventions are the cornerstone of drug treatment. A large evidence base exists for psycho-social interventions for established legal and illegal drugs, along with guidance for implementation.[20][21][22][23] It is beyond the scope of this book to comprehensively review these interventions.

At present, there is very little evidence available to guide the clinician in managing people harmfully using club drugs and NPS. In the absence of this evidence, it is suggested that existing psycho-social interventions for 'traditional' drugs are used. Research into the effectiveness of these interventions is a priority.

Figures 5.1–5.4 provide a broad overview of acute and chronic adverse effects of club drugs and NPS alongside their clinical management. The following chapters will discuss each drug group in more detail.

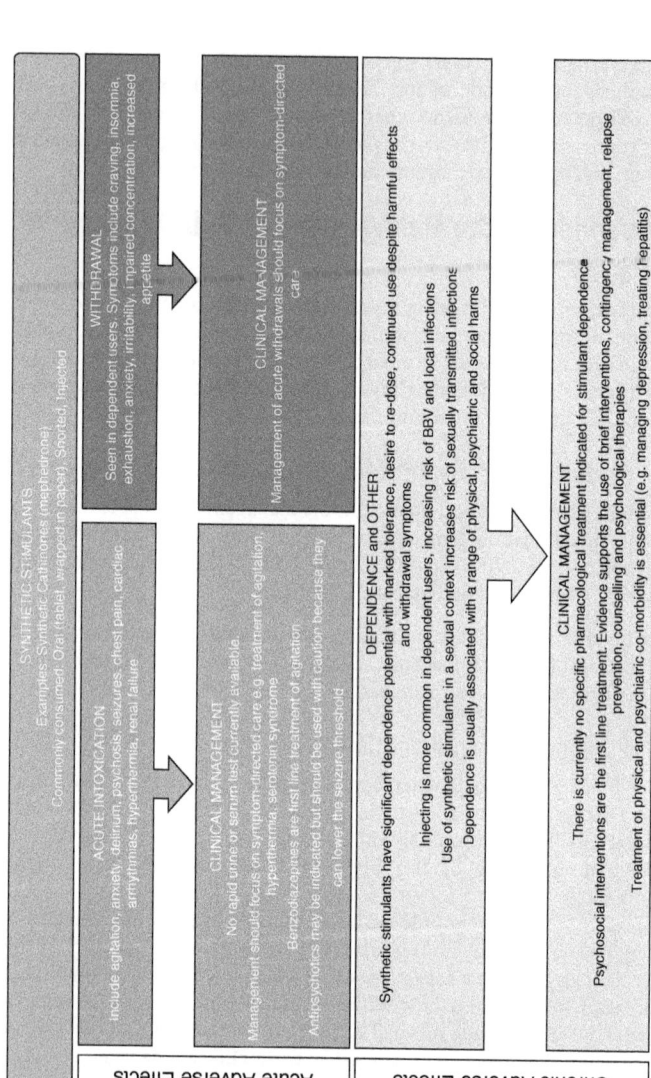

Figure 5.1 Acute and chronic harms of stimulants

The content within the figure reads:

SYNTHETIC STIMULANTS
Examples: Synthetic Cathinones (mephedrone)
Commonly consumed: Oral (tablet, wrapped in paper), Snorted, Injected

Acute Adverse Effects

ACUTE INTOXICATION
Include agitation, anxiety, delirium, psychosis, seizures, chest pain, cardiac arrhythmias, hyperthermia, renal failure

CLINICAL MANAGEMENT
No rapid urine or serum test currently available.
Management should focus on symptom-directed care e.g. treatment of agitation hyperthermia, serotonin syndrome
Benzodiazepines are first line treatment of agitation
Antipsychotics may be indicated but should be used with caution because they can lower the seizure threshold

WITHDRAWAL
Seen in dependent users. Symptoms include craving, insomnia, exhaustion, anxiety, irritability, impaired concentration, increased appetite

CLINICAL MANAGEMENT
Management of acute withdrawals should focus on symptom-directed care

Chronic Adverse Effects

DEPENDENCE and OTHER
Synthetic stimulants have significant dependence potential with marked tolerance, desire to re-dose, continued use despite harmful effects and withdrawal symptoms
Injecting is more common in dependent users, increasing risk of BBV and local infections
Use of synthetic stimulants in a sexual context increases risk of sexually transmitted infections
Dependence is usually associated with a range of physical, psychiatric and social harms

CLINICAL MANAGEMENT
There is currently no specific pharmacological treatment indicated for stimulant dependence
Psychosocial interventions are the first line treatment. Evidence supports the use of brief interventions, contingency management, relapse prevention, counselling and psychological therapies
Treatment of physical and psychiatric co-morbidity is essential (e.g. managing depression, treating hepatitis)

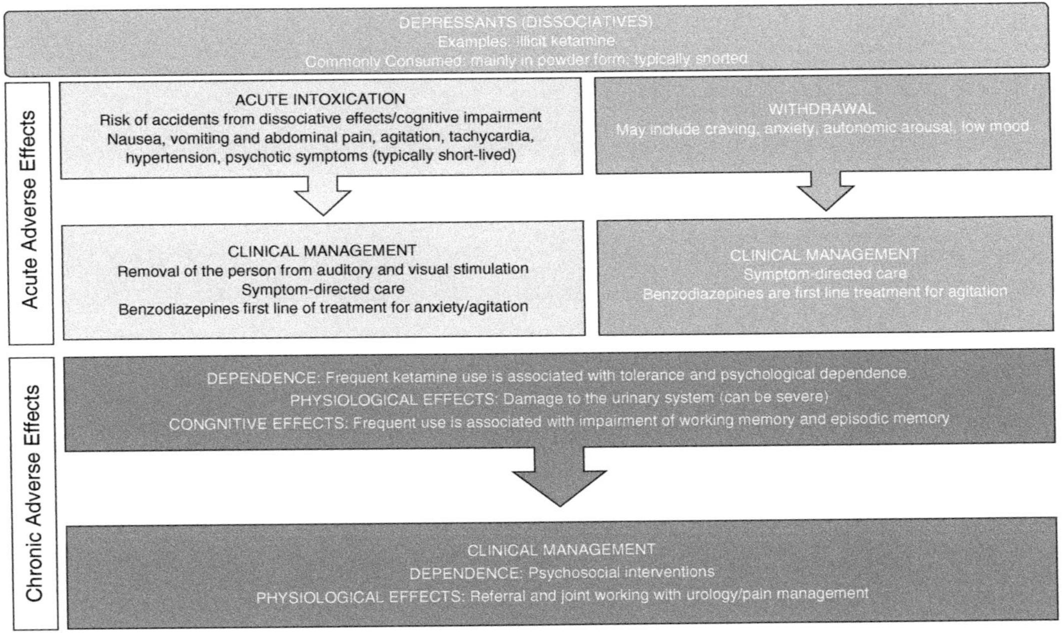
DEPRESSANTS (DISSOCIATIVES)
Examples: illicit ketamine
Commonly Consumed: mainly in powder form; typically snorted
Acute Adverse Effects
ACUTE INTOXICATION
Risk of accidents from dissociative effects/cognitive impairment
Nausea, vomiting and abdominal pain, agitation, tachycardia, hypertension, psychotic symptoms (typically short-lived)
CLINICAL MANAGEMENT
Removal of the person from auditory and visual stimulation
Symptom-directed care
Benzodiazepines first line of treatment for anxiety/agitation
WITHDRAWAL
May include craving, anxiety, autonomic arousal, low mood
CLINICAL MANAGEMENT
Symptom-directed care
Benzodiazepines are first line treatment for agitation
Chronic Adverse Effects
DEPENDENCE: Frequent ketamine use is associated with tolerance and psychological dependence.
PHYSIOLOGICAL EFFECTS: Damage to the urinary system (can be severe)
CONGNITIVE EFFECTS: Frequent use is associated with impairment of working memory and episodic memory
CLINICAL MANAGEMENT
DEPENDENCE: Psychosocial interventions
PHYSIOLOGICAL EFFECTS: Referral and joint working with urology/pain management

Figure 5.2 Acute and chronic harms of depressants

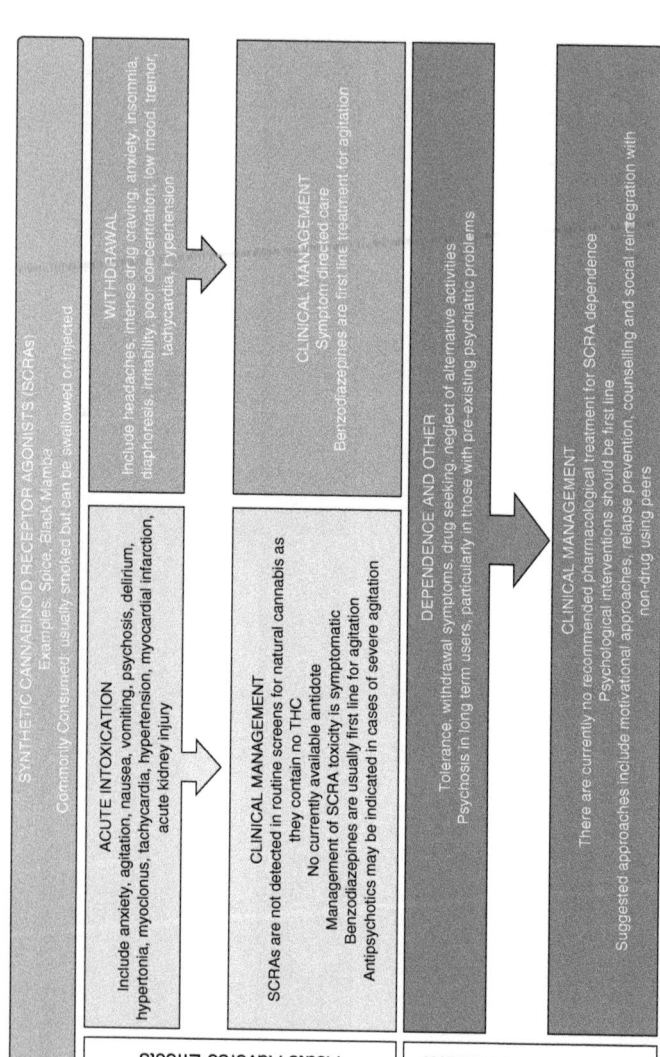

Figure 5.3 Acute and chronic harms of synthetic cannabinoid receptor agonists (SCRAs)

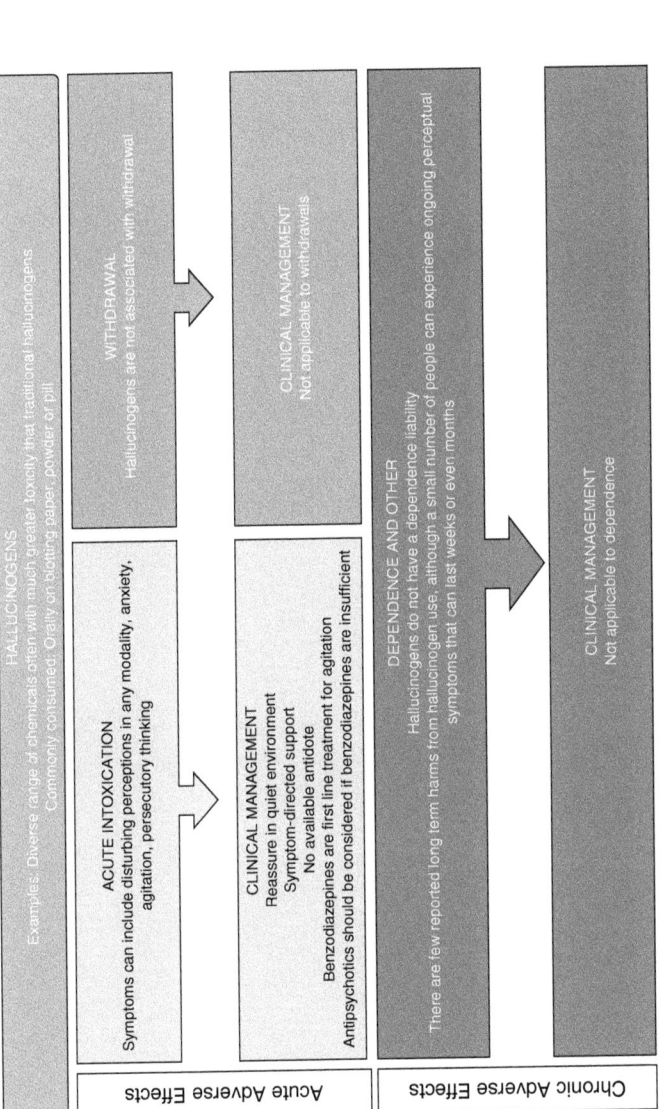

HALLUCINOGENS

Examples: Diverse range of chemicals often with much greater toxicity that traditional hallucinogens
Commonly consumed: Orally on blotting paper, powder or pill

Acute Adverse Effects

ACUTE INTOXICATION
Symptoms can include disturbing perceptions in any modality, anxiety, agitation, persecutory thinking

CLINICAL MANAGEMENT
Reassure in quiet environment
Symptom-directed support
No available antidote
Benzodiazepines are first line treatment for agitation
Antipsychotics should be considered if benzodiazepines are insufficient

WITHDRAWAL
Hallucinogens are not associated with withdrawal

CLINICAL MANAGEMENT
Not applicable to withdrawals

Chronic Adverse Effects

DEPENDENCE AND OTHER
Hallucinogens do not have a dependence liability
There are few reported long term harms from hallucinogen use, although a small number of people can experience ongoing perceptual symptoms that can last weeks or even months

CLINICAL MANAGEMENT
Not applicable to dependence

Figure 5.4 Acute and chronic harms of hallucinogens

Chapter

Stimulant Drugs: Introduction

6.1 Introduction and Brief Pharmacology of Stimulant Drugs

Stimulant drugs form the largest category of recreational drugs and include cocaine and amphetamine-type stimulants (ATS).

Stimulant drugs belong to a variety of different chemical groups. They stimulate the central nervous system by increasing the availability of key neurotransmitters at brain receptor sites, particularly dopamine, noradrenaline and serotonin. Stimulant drugs increase the levels of active neurotransmitters by increasing their release from pre-synaptic neurons or by inhibiting the reuptake of these neurotransmitters. Some stimulants do both.

The extent to which a specific drug elevates the levels of noradrenaline, dopamine and serotonin will determine its psychoactive effect, including desired effect.

- Drugs that increase active dopamine enhance pleasure and can lead to euphoria. They are also more likely to increase a desire to re-dose (e.g. cocaine).
- Drugs that increase active noradrenaline will be less euphoric, but increase alertness and may cause anxiety. They are also more likely to have cardiac effects (e.g. amphetamine).
- Drugs that increase serotonin activity can have empathy-inducing effects and are sometimes referred to as 'empathogenic' drugs (e.g. MDMA).

Different types of stimulants will therefore operate differently. Cocaine increases the activity of neurotransmitters in the central and peripheral nervous systems by blocking reuptake transporters of dopamine, noradrenaline and serotonin. Amphetamine-type substances, on the other hand, will generally increase the pre-synaptic release of dopamine.

6.2 Desired Effects of Stimulants by User

When a drug user consumes a stimulant drug, the desired effects typically include increased energy, mood enhancement, euphoria, mental clarity, improved concentration, improved sociability, and in some cases empathy-inducing and pro-sexual effects. Stimulants can also reduce appetite and the need for sleep.

6.3 Adverse Health Harms of Stimulants

Stimulant use is associated with a range of acute and longer-term health effects, including sympathomimetic effects, serotonin syndrome and mental health problems including psychosis.

Most stimulants have broadly similar adverse health effects. However, there are differences in the extent to which a particular drug is associated with particular adverse effects; these will be highlighted later in sections on specific substances.

6.4 Acute Health Harms of Stimulants

6.4.1 The Features of Acute Toxicity

Acute **toxicity** – or 'overdose', as many drug users may describe it – can lead to a range of acute psychiatric (Box 6.1) and physiological harms (Box 6.2).

Box 6.1 Psychiatric and Psychological Effects of Acute Stimulant Intoxication

Stimulants are characterised by their acute effects on mental state. Agitation is a common adverse effect of stimulant intoxication. Stimulants in general are more likely to induce psychosis and a range of mental health problems than other illicit drugs.[24]

Features of acute intoxication can include:
- Rapid mood changes, including euphoria, dysphoria and depression with suicidal thinking
- Delirium
- Agitation, anxiety, restlessness, aggressiveness
- Psychosis, including persecutory thinking (overvalued and delusional thinking) and hallucinations (may be in any modality, but typically auditory and/or tactile)

Box 6.2 Physiological Effects of Stimulant Intoxication

Stimulants have sympathomimetic and vasoconstrictor effects.

Stimulants increase heart rate, blood pressure and breathing rates; constrict blood vessels; dilate pupils; and release glucose and lipids into the bloodstream. Stimulants are characterised by their neurotoxicity and cardiotoxicity.

Features of stimulant intoxication include:[25]

- diaphoresis, tachycardia, hypertension, chest pain, myocardial infarction, cardiomyopathy[26] and cerebrovascular accidents[27]
- seizures
- hyperthermia, which can result in complications including rhabdomyolysis, acute renal failure, disseminated intravascular coagulation and multiple organ failure[28] [29]
- serotonin syndrome, especially where more than one serotonergic agent has been used (see Section 6.6)
- neuroleptic malignant syndrome

6.5 Management of Acute Harms of Stimulants

The management of acute stimulant toxicity is symptomatic and supportive as no antidotes exist.

Supportive treatment is dependent on a patient's specific presentation and typically includes exclusion of underlying pathology and the use of benzodiazepines for agitation.

TOXBASE® suggests that basic management should include:

- maintenance of airway and ventilation
- monitoring of vital signs
- initial investigations should include papillary blood glucose, ECG, blood testing for FBC, U&Es, LTFs, CK and INR.

Other causes of the clinical presentation, such as infection, hypoxia and hypoglycaemia, should be excluded.

Agitation can be treated by nursing the patient in a low-stimulus environment and administration of benzodiazepines, provided there is no impairment of respiratory function.

The benefit of gastric decontamination is uncertain. Consider oral-activated charcoal if illicit stimulant has been ingested within one hour.

For a patient in cardiac arrest, resuscitation should be considered for at least 1 hour. Prolonged resuscitation may be appropriate as recovery with good neurological outcome may occur. See TOXBASE* for more details.

6.6 Serotonin Syndrome

Serotonin syndrome, sometimes known as serotonin poisoning, is a potentially life-threatening syndrome resulting from excess serotonergic agonism of CNS and peripheral serotonergic receptors.[30] [31]

There may be considerable overlap between hyperthermia and serotonin syndrome. Serotonin syndrome can be a trigger for uncontrolled hyperthermia, but hyperthermia can also occur without serotonin syndrome.[32]

Serotonin syndrome is associated with a wide range of illicit drugs and prescribed medications such as selective serotonin reuptake inhibitors (SSRIs), monoamine oxidase inhibitors (MAOIs), serotonin-noradrenaline reuptake inhibitors (SNRIs) and tricyclic antidepressants, among others.

Large or repeated doses of stimulants increase serotonin release. The simultaneous use of multiple stimulants increases the risk of serotonin toxicity, as does dehydration and hyperthermia.

6.6.1 Features of Serotonin Syndrome

Serotonin syndrome has three classic features[33] but not all three will necessarily manifest in all patients:

- neuromuscular abnormalities (including hyperreflexia, inducible, ocular or spontaneous clonus, peripheral hypertonicity and shivering)
- autonomic hyperactivity (including tachycardia, hyperpyrexia, mydriasis, diaphoresis and diarrhoea)
- mental state changes (agitation and delirium)

6.6.2 Assessment of Serotonin Syndrome

The features of serotonin syndrome typically occur within minutes to hours after drug exposure.

The clinical symptoms are on a spectrum of severity, from mild to life threatening.[34] [35] [36] [37] Clinical features may include the following:

Mild:
- Patients can be afebrile
- Shivering
- Diaphoresis
- Mydriasis
- Tachycardia

Moderate:

- Agitation or hypervigilance
- Slightly pressured speech
- Hyperactive bowel sounds
- Severe diaphoresis
- Tachycardia and hypertension
- Hyperthermia (40°C is common)
- There may be repetitive rotation of the head, with the neck held in moderate extension
- Hyperreflexia and clonus, especially in lower extremities
- Horizontal ocular clonus

Severe:

- Severe hypertension and tachycardia that might deteriorate abruptly into frank shock
- Agitated delirium
- Muscle rigidity and hypertonicity, and increase in muscle tone (usually considerably greater in lower extremities than upper)
- Muscle hyperactivity may produce a core temperature of more than 41.1°C in some cases
- Metabolic acidosis, rhabdomyolysis, elevated levels of serum aminotransferase and creatinine, seizures, renal failure, disseminated intravascular coagulopathy

There are no laboratory tests to confirm the diagnosis of serotonin syndrome; however, a number of diagnostic approaches/tools for serotonin syndrome are available.

Formalised diagnostic approaches to serotonin syndrome include the 'Hunter Serotonin Toxicity Criteria: decision rules'.[31]

History and physical examination should include:

- The quantity and type of drugs ingested
- The evolution and rate of progression of symptoms
- Presence of tremor, clonus or akathisia with no additional extrapyramidal signs.

Clonus (spontaneous, inducible and ocular) is considered the most important sign indicating developing serotonin syndrome.

6.6.3   Management of Serotonin Syndrome

Most cases of serotonin syndrome are self-limiting and may be treated with supportive care and by refraining from further use of serotonergic drugs. Most mild cases will resolve spontaneously within 24 hours.

Initial treatment should include cessation of all serotonergic agents, monitoring of vital signs and initial investigations (capillary blood sugar, ECG, routine blood screen). Fluid intake and urine output should be monitored to ensure appropriate hydration.

Other causes of the clinical presentation, such as infection, hypoxia and hypoglycaemia, should be excluded.

Agitation can be treated by nursing the patient in a low-stimulus environment and administration of benzodiazepines, provided there is no impairment of respiratory function.

Serotonin syndrome can potentially be very severe. Patients with moderate or severe cases of serotonin syndrome require hospitalisation. In some cases clinical symptoms may persist for longer, particularly in cases involving serotonergic drugs with long duration of action or active metabolites.

People with drug-related serotonin syndrome often present to hospitals with advanced symptoms because some of the early, mild signs of the syndrome are perceived as normal drug effects.

In serious cases, TOXBASE® suggests the consideration of the 5-HT$_{2A}$ antagonists cyproheptadine and chlorpromazine. See TOXBASE® for further details.

6.7 Health Harms from Repeated Use of Stimulants

The persistent use of stimulants can lead to a number of adverse physical and psychiatric health consequences. Their severity will depend on the frequency of dosing, quantity consumed, length of consumption and route of administration.

6.7.1 Physical Harms Associated with Prolonged Use of Stimulants

Physical Harm Associated with Mode of Use

Insufflation: Snorting powder cocaine or other stimulants regularly can lead to loss of smell, nosebleeds, problems with swallowing, hoarseness, and an overall irritation of the nasal septum leading to chronic inflammation, rhinorrhoea or even perforation.

Injecting: viral and bacterial infections, vein damage

Smoking: cough, asthma, respiratory distress and lung infections

Ingestion by mouth: severe bowel ulceration and necrosis resulting from reduced blood flow.

6.7.2 Psychiatric Harms Associated with Prolonged Use of Stimulants

Dependence
Repeated use of stimulants can result in physiological and/or psychological dependence. The risk of dependence depends on both drug factors (pattern of use, differing dependence risk of particular stimulants) and characteristics of the individual consuming the drug (genetic vulnerability; physical, mental and social morbidity).

Stimulant Withdrawal
When stimulants are used regularly, cessation or even a reduction in the quantity used may precipitate withdrawal symptoms.

Three phases of stimulant withdrawal are recognised.

- **'Crash'**: typically commences following abrupt cessation of heavy use of stimulants. Features include exhaustion, fatigue, agitation and irritability, depression, muscle ache, akathisia and sleep disturbances (typically increased sleep, although insomnia or restless sleep may occur). The 'crash' typically commences 12–24 hours after last stimulant use and subsides within 2–4 days.
- **'Withdrawal'**: characterised by a strong desire to use the drug (cravings). Other features include fluctuating mood and energy levels, alternating between irritability, restlessness, anxiety, agitation and fatigue. This phase typically commences 2–4 days after last use, peaks in severity over 7–10 days and then subsides over 2–4 weeks.
- **'Extinction'**: gradual resumption of normal mood with episodic fluctuations in mood and energy levels, alternating between irritability, restlessness, anxiety, agitation, fatigue, lack of energy, episodic cravings and disturbed sleep. This may last weeks to months.

Prolonged use of stimulants can also lead to a range of other mental health problems, including anxiety and mood disorders, persecutory thinking and, albeit rarely, psychosis.

6.8 Management of Harms from Repeated Use of Stimulants

6.8.1 Management of Physical Harms
Physical harms associated with prolonged use of stimulants typically resolve with cessation of use, although some harms, such as nasal perforation,

acquisition of blood-borne viruses and lung damage, require further medical intervention.

6.8.2 Management of Stimulant Dependence and Withdrawal Symptoms

Pharmacological Interventions

At present there are no pharmacological treatments for stimulant dependence that have proven efficacy, although a number of promising research studies are taking place on new medications. Withdrawal symptoms should be managed symptomatically – for example, with management of insomnia and agitation.

Psycho-Social Interventions

Behavioural therapies and psycho-social interventions are currently the main effective treatment for stimulant dependence. There is currently no research consensus indicating that one particular psycho-social intervention is more effective than another.

Stimulant Drugs: Cocaine

7.1 Introduction and Brief Pharmacology

Cocaine is one of the most commonly used illicit drugs in the UK and globally, with an estimated 18.1 million people having used it globally in the last year according to the 2019 World Drug Report.[2] In England and Wales, when estimating drug use in the last year, powder cocaine was second only to cannabis for adults aged 16–59 (2.9% in the 2018/19 survey, equating to around 976,000 people). Powder cocaine was also the third most commonly used drug among young adults aged 16–24 (6.2%, or around 395,000 young adults), following cannabis and nitrous oxide.[38]

Cocaine stimulates the sympathetic nervous system primarily by increasing the availability of monoamine neurotransmitters (dopamine, noradrenaline and serotonin) in the central and peripheral nervous system by blocking their reuptake. In addition, cocaine can affect other neurotransmitter systems, including the endogenous opioid system.

7.2 Modes of Use

Cocaine is absorbed readily through all mucosae. Cocaine powder is most commonly insufflated (snorted), but can be smoked, rubbed on the gums, or used intravenously or rectally.

7.3 Desired Effects by User

The desired effects of cocaine use are feelings of increased energy, alertness and intense euphoria, as well as a decrease in tiredness, appetite and sleep.

7.4 Acute Health Harms

The general acute adverse health effects of cocaine are similar to those of other stimulants. The acute harms associated with the use of cocaine can be due to sympathomimetic effects of cocaine or due to the effects of cutting agents.

7.4.1 Cardio-Toxic Effects

- Significant toxic effects on the heart and cardiovascular system, including being a powerful vasoconstrictor.[39]

  - Cardiovascular and circulatory disorders can include acute coronary ischaemia and infarction, arrhythmia, myocarditis, pulmonary oedema, pulmonary infarction, pulmonary hypertension, mesenteric ischaemia or infarction. Cocaine can increase the risk of thrombotic and non-thrombotic acute coronary syndrome and arterial dissection.

- Cerebrovascular disorders and neurological impairment, including cerebrovascular accident (stroke), and status epilepticus.
- Reduction of blood flow in the gastrointestinal tract, which can lead to ulceration and perforation.[40]
- Associated renal, genito-urinary and obstetric disorders, including acute renal failure (mediated by rhabdomyolysis or direct toxicity), testicular infarction, placental abruption, spontaneous abortion and premature birth.

Cocaine is particularly cardio-toxic, especially when used with alcohol. The combination of cocaine and ethanol produces a significant synergistic depression of ventricular contraction and relaxation which exceeds the arithmetic sum of the depressive effects of either cocaine or ethanol alone. The combination of cocaine and ethanol also result in the in vivo formation of cocaethylene, a more cardio-toxic substance with a longer period of action.[41] Co-ingestion of cocaine and alcohol has also been reported to increase the likelihood of hospitalisation.[42]

7.5 Case 1 Cocaine User with Chest Pain

Presenting Complaint and History
Eddie is a 28-year-old solicitor living with his girlfriend of two years. He is a regular drinker, with a decade-long pattern of consuming around 20 Standard Alcohol Units (SAU) a week in two binges. Approximately twice a year, Eddie uses 'a little bit of cocaine' during an alcohol binge. The cocaine is supplied to him by a 'friend of a friend'.

The night of his presentation to the Emergency Department, Eddie had been out with friends celebrating his birthday. He had consumed four pints of beer before snorting 'three lines' of cocaine, which a friend had bought him as a birthday present. Immediately, Eddie felt alert and euphoric, but also experienced his heart 'racing'. Previous cocaine use had also caused this symptom for

Eddie, but it usually resolved after a few minutes. This time, however, after 5 minutes, his heart 'got faster and faster' and Eddie experienced a 'pounding' in his chest. He began to feel anxious, and a few minutes later experienced a sharp tightness across his chest. Eddie was now highly distressed and felt that he was having a heart attack. He asked his friends to call an ambulance.

Assessment
On arrival at the Emergency Room, Eddie was agitated and distressed, tachycardic (120 b/min) and hypertensive (162/104). An ECG confirmed sinus tachycardia but showed no signs of ischaemia. A chest x-ray and routine blood tests including a troponin and venous blood gas were unremarkable except for a slightly raised Gamma GT and blood alcohol level.

Management
Symptomatic management was commenced, including diazepam 5mg, oral analgesia and reassurance. He was also given two puffs of sublingual GTN.

After taking the diazepam, Eddie began to feel calmer. His heart rate and blood pressure reduced to within normal levels and the chest pain abated.

Advice was given to Eddie on the risks of cocaine and alcohol, particularly when mixed together. It was explained that his blood tests showed the effects of excessive alcohol consumption and there followed a discussion on what constitutes a safe limit of alcohol use.

The offer of a referral to substance misuse services was made.

Eddie was discharged.

Key Learning
Cocaine is a common cause of chest pain in adults, secondary to the vasoconstrictive effects on vessels.

Combining cocaine and alcohol increases the risks, partly due to the formation of cocaethyline – a cardio-toxic byproduct of co-ingestion.

Management of cocaine-induced chest pain typically involves the exclusion of acute harm such as myocardial infarction. Local treatment protocols should be used as indicated.

If acute harms are excluded then symptomatic management is indicated.

7.6 Management of Acute Health Harms

The management of acute adverse effects of cocaine should follow the same protocols as for other stimulants. Particular attention should be given to the assessment and management of cardiac harms, which are generally more common with cocaine use than with other stimulants.

7.7 Health Harms from Prolonged Use

- Repeated cocaine use has been associated with a range of physical and psychiatric harms similar to stimulants in general. These include psychiatric effects, such as dependence and mood disorders, and physical effects, such as nose bleeds and hepatocellular damage. Other harms include musculoskeletal disorders and movement disorders.

7.8 Case 2 Cocaine Dependence

Presenting Complaint/History

Angela is a 28-year-old antique dealer who runs a business with her husband, Jake. They have been together for 8 years, and during that time have both used a range of psychoactive substances, including alcohol, cocaine, ketamine and MDMA.

Over the last two years, Angela's use of cocaine has increased significantly. She seeks out the drug at parties and particularly enjoys the strong euphoric effect. Angela thinks her cocaine use is 'just fun' and consumes around half a gram, once a week, 'the same as everyone else'.

In the last year Jake has become increasingly concerned about Angela's drug use and has repeatedly asked her to cut down. He believes that Angela is using much more cocaine than their friends and tries to stay by her side at parties to 'keep an eye' on her use. Angela is irritated by Jake when he suggests she is using excessively, telling him he is 'boring' and 'uptight'. To avoid confrontation with Jake, Angela has contacted an acquaintance who has agreed to sell her cocaine whenever she wants it. Angela now uses cocaine less at parties, which pleases Jake, but has instead started using on her own at home without Jake's knowledge. She feels the euphoric effect is even more powerful when using alone and is careful to hide her use from Jake by waiting until he is out of the house or away on business.

In the last six months, Angela has used cocaine on most days. She takes a supply to the shop the couple own and uses small amounts throughout the day. Angela has noticed that the euphoric effect of cocaine has diminished and as a result has needed to increase her consumption to experience even modestly elevated mood. She is now consuming around 1 gram a day, 6–7 days a week. Angela rationalises that this increase in dose is because the cocaine she is supplied with is of poorer quality. Although Jake is unaware of Angela's increased cocaine use, he has noticed that she is moody, frequently irritable with him and has been spending more money, which she told him is to purchase new stock for the shop.

Although she has successfully concealed her cocaine consumption, Angela is now worried about her use. She is spending more and more money on cocaine and does not know how to hide this from Jake or her friends. She has stopped attending parties and also avoids social engagements as she thinks people will be able 'to tell what I am up to'. Angela has also begun to feel physically unwell, with persistent lethargy, low mood and outbursts of anger. She has also started to crave cocaine, something she has never experienced before. Angela has made several unsuccessful attempts to reduce her cocaine use and has deleted her dealer's number on four occasions, only to find a way of re-contacting him.

Angela feels too embarrassed to talk to Jake and is worried about his reaction to the money she has spent from the business account.

One day, Angela feels too unwell to go to work. Desperate to use cocaine, but also distressed by the control the drug seems to have taken over her life, she tells Jake everything and asks for help. Jake is shocked and, not knowing what to do, looks up the address of the local drug service, makes an appointment for Angela and accompanies her to the assessment.

Assessment

At assessment, Angela is tearful and distressed. She has not used cocaine for 48 hours and is strongly craving the drug. Angela explains that she has a strong family history of addiction, including her father who was a pathological gambler, her mother who is alcohol dependent and a maternal uncle who died of a heroin overdose. Angela fulfils the ICD-11 criteria for cocaine dependence, with symptoms including significant drug craving, difficulty controlling her level of use, cocaine withdrawal symptoms, tolerance, persistent use despite harmful effects and a loss of interest in other activities.

Angela also describes other symptoms, including low mood, loss of pleasure, reduced energy, poor concentration and reduced appetite with weight loss. It is unclear whether these symptoms are a direct effect of the cocaine use or represent a co-existing depressive disorder.

At assessment, Angela identifies her goal as complete abstinence from cocaine use.

Management

Angela attends weekly key-working sessions aimed at acquiring a better understanding of the situation and to help her develop psychological strategies to manage her cravings for cocaine, an approach known as 'relapse prevention'. She completes a craving diary and a number of other exercises to understand what she feels are the benefits and drawbacks of her use. Angela also attends Cocaine Anonymous, where she meets other people experiencing similar problems.

After a month in treatment, Angela has not used any cocaine. To her surprise, the depressive symptoms have subsided and she has not experienced any further episodes of anger or cravings for the drug. Angela now has a sponsor at Cocaine Anonymous who she meets with regularly to discuss remaining abstinent. She continues to attend the clinic for support, and her husband has also met with staff to understand how he can best help Angela.

Key Learning

Dependence typically develops slowly, over months or even years.

Many people with dependence will deny that they have a problem and will not see the need for treatment.

The symptoms of dependence can be difficult to distinguish from other psychiatric symptoms, such as depressive episodes and anxiety disorder.

7.9 Management of Cocaine Dependence and Withdrawal Symptoms

As mentioned in Chapter 6, there are currently no proven pharmacological treatments for cocaine dependence. Psycho-social interventions are currently recommended, although the evidence does not support one particular intervention over another.

Chapter

8

Stimulant Drugs: Amphetamine-Type Stimulants

8.1 Introduction and Brief Psychopharmacology

Amphetamine-type stimulants (ATS) refer to a group of stimulant drugs whose principal members include amphetamine and methamphetamine, but also include a range of other substances, such as MDMA. ATS are the second most popular group of illegal drugs after cannabis.[2]

A diverse range of other substances also fall into this group, and ATS include both well-established and new psychoactive substances with primarily stimulant effects. Indeed, a significant proportion of NPS reported to the UNODC are ATS. According to the World Drug Report (2019)[1] the number of stimulant NPS identified between 2009 and 2017 increased more than fourfold, from 48 substances in 2009 to a peak of 206 in 2015. In most years, stimulant NPS have been the largest group of NPS identified, followed by synthetic cannabinoids. More than a third of all NPS identified since 2009 are stimulants. A total of 26 out of the 79 new substances that were identified and reported for the first time in 2017 were stimulants.

The term 'amphetamine-type stimulants' (ATS) is used to refer to groups of substances or amphetamine analogues with stimulant effects, such as phenethylamines (e.g. MDMA), and methcathinone and other synthetic cathinones (e.g. mephedrone).

ATS in general increase the release of dopamine, in contrast to stimulants such as cocaine, which prevents dopamine reuptake. As a result, the effects of ATS typically last longer than those of cocaine.

The different ATS share common properties; however, their effects must not be seen as homogeneous. ATS sit on a continuum of stimulant, hallucinogenic and euphoriant effects; indeed, many have a combination of all these effects. Some stimulants, such as MDMA, have distinct social and emotional effects, leading some to propose that they should be classed as 'entactogens' or 'empathogens'. Some ATS are reported to have a pro-sexual effect. ATS also differ in the level of their dependence liability.

Chapters 9, 10 and 11 will examine the three most commonly used ATS: methamphetamine, MDMA and the cathinone mephedrone.

Chapter 9

Stimulant Drugs: Methamphetamine

9.1 Introduction and Brief Pharmacology

Methamphetamine is a member of the phenethylamine family. It is a potent psychomotor stimulant with physical and psychological effects. It is typically described as a more potent, longer-lasting stimulant than amphetamine, is highly lipophilic, and, in comparison with amphetamine at similar doses, it crosses the blood–brain barrier more easily.

9.2 Modes of Use

Methamphetamine is a synthetic drug that is usually manufactured in illegal laboratories. It is produced as a powder, in tablet form or as crystals that look like shards of glass.

The most common form of methamphetamine found in the UK at the time of writing is a hydrochloride salt, which is typically produced as a white or off-white bitter-tasting powder, or as purer crystals that are soluble in water. It has been reported that it is sometimes produced as tablets, which carry logos similar to those on ecstasy tablets.

In the UK methamphetamine is currently mainly smoked, but it is also snorted, injected intravenously (known as 'slamming' among men who have sex with men (MSM) in the UK) or inserted rectally.

At the time of writing, methamphetamine use in the UK is mainly concentrated among gay men and MSM (see Section 9.9)

9.3 Desired Effects by User

Desired effects include increased alertness, energy and confidence, focused attention, decreased appetite and euphoria. In methamphetamine-naïve individuals, acute doses can improve cognitive processing.

Methamphetamine can increase sexual drive and reduce sexual inhibition. It is sometimes consumed in a sexual context, especially by gay men and other MSM, where this is sometimes referred to as 'chemsex'.

9.4 Acute Health Harms

The physiological acute harms of methamphetamine are similar overall to those of other stimulants described in Chapter 6.

Notable harms reported with methamphetamine include psychiatric effects, particularly methamphetamine-induced psychosis. The aetiology is poorly understood; however, methamphetamine-induced psychotic disorder has been associated with both acute intoxication and chronic, high-dose and continuous use of methamphetamine.[43]

The association between methamphetamine use and mental health problems (including psychosis) is well documented, especially where there is frequent use.[44] Methamphetamine intoxication can result in symptoms such as persecutory thinking, delusions and auditory, visual and tactile hallucinations.[45] The clinical presentation can be indistinguishable from an acute episode of paranoid schizophrenia.[46] Acute intoxication is often associated with significant mood disturbances.

Symptoms usually remit as the effects of methamphetamine subside, but some people may develop psychosis that lasts weeks or months after stopping methamphetamine. Psychotic symptoms may prove to be refractory to antipsychotic medication.[47]

Persistent, heavy use of methamphetamine can also be associated with methamphetamine-induced psychosis.[48]

People who use methamphetamine will have different vulnerabilities to psychosis, but psychotic symptoms are more prevalent among people who use methamphetamine on a regular basis.[44] The most consistent correlates of psychotic symptoms are increased frequency of methamphetamine use and dependence on methamphetamine.[49] Other predictors, such as genetic vulnerability, may also play a role.[45]

There is also some evidence that methamphetamine can exacerbate existing mental health problems.[24] Dysphoria, depression, anxiety, suicidal ideation and cognitive deficits often co-occur in people using methamphetamine. One study suggested that people who experience depressive symptoms and use methamphetamine may have a poorer prognosis for both conditions and may experience worse treatment outcomes.[50]

9.5 Case 3 Methamphetamine-Induced Psychosis

Presenting Complaint/History

Fabian is a 45-year-old gay man; he works as an architect and lives with his partner, Eric. Fabian had never used any illicit drugs until, at the age of 43, he met Eric, who introduced him to methamphetamine. Initially, Fabian and Eric only used methamphetamine when together to enhance sexual pleasure, and only consumed the drug by smoking. Fabian was aware that methamphetamine could be addictive, but was reassured by Eric that they would be careful. Eric had used methamphetamine for more than a decade, solely for sexual enhancement, and denied any problems with his use at any point. Fabian never purchased or prepared the drug, leaving this to Eric.

Fabian found the effects of methamphetamine 'amazing'. When smoking the drug he experienced an almost instantaneous 'high' with intense euphoria and alertness. Although the drug improved his sex life with Eric, Fabian also realised that methamphetamine made him feel 'focused and motivated'. He found the drug 'moreish' and after a few months experimented with using the methamphetamine on his own, not for its sexual effects but to motivate himself during busy periods at work. If he smoked a small amount of methamphetamine before going to work, he felt alert, energised and produced work that was 'twice as good, twice as fast'.

Fabian increasingly used methamphetamine to help him meet work deadlines. He mentioned this to Eric, who warned him to be careful and reluctantly agreed to provide Fabian with the name of his dealer. Fabian's use gradually escalated to around once a week, although he described only benefits and no harmful effects.

A month ago, Fabian became worried that colleagues at work were planning to have him sacked and were 'plotting against me'. He felt that they were building a case for dismissal against him and would see them talking to each other in the office in a suspicious manner. He wondered whether they were checking his emails and repeatedly changed his passwords. He spoke to Eric, who reassured him that he was imagining it, but Fabian became increasingly concerned. He threw away his laptop because he thought it had been 'bugged' and bought a new one, but after a few weeks he threw that away as well. On a number of occasions, Eric discovered Fabian re-setting his mobile phone to factory setting and changing the SIM card in the middle of the night, 'just to make sure' his colleagues had not installed surveillance software without his knowledge.

Eric became increasingly worried about Fabian and asked him to stop using methamphetamine as he thought this might be the cause of the persecutory thinking. Fabian refused, saying it was the only thing that made him feel 'normal'. Eric refused to buy any more methamphetamine and contacted the dealer to ask him to stop supplying Fabian. Fabian quickly found a new dealer to supply him. He was now smoking methamphetamine every day in an attempt 'to cope'.

Three days ago, Fabian stopped going to work as he thought he might be attacked by his colleagues. He had seen an item on the news about a police crackdown on drugs and was convinced that the news channel was running it as a personal warning that something dreadful was about to happen to him. Fabian told Eric that he feared for his life and that he knew that if he went to work his work colleagues would try to murder him. When Eric tried to reassure

Fabian, he ran to his bedroom and barricaded the door, shouting that he could no longer trust anyone.

Not knowing what else to do, Eric called his GP, who arranged a Mental Health Act assessment with the police in attendance. Fabian was brought to the local psychiatric hospital under section for further assessment.

Assessment

Fabian presented as suspicious and hostile. He refused to answer any questions but asked for 'all the secret cameras to be turned off'.

Eric stated that to his knowledge Fabian had no previous history of physical or mental health problems, and none in the family. Aside from methamphetamine there was no other drug or alcohol use.

A provisional diagnosis of methamphetamine-induced psychosis was made and a plan drawn up to observe him as an inpatient.

Management

On the ward Fabian initially said he felt 'safe', but was very guarded with staff. There continued to be evidence of persecutory thinking of delusional intensity but no obvious auditory or visual hallucinations. Routine bloods were taken which were unremarkable. A urine drug screen revealed only methamphetamine.

After 24 hours, Fabian became very agitated and verbally aggressive with staff. He demanded to leave the hospital, stating that he needed to take methamphetamine 'to get well'. He was offered diazepam and night sedation, both of which he accepted, resulting in him feeling calmer and sleeping well.

Over the next ten days, Fabian's psychotic symptoms began to improve. He began to question whether some of his suspicions were correct and his interaction with staff became much less guarded. He was regularly visited by Eric, who suggested to Fabian that methamphetamine was the likely cause of his symptoms.

After ten days, Fabian was asymptomatic and had full insight. He accepted that methamphetamine use had caused his symptoms and vowed never to use this or any other drug again.

Key Learning

Methamphetamine, more than other stimulants, appears to precipitate psychotic symptoms in some users.

Clinical presentation can be indistinguishable from other forms of psychosis including an acute episode of paranoid schizophrenia.

A urine drug screen is indicated is all such presentations, and well as investigations to exclude organic causes of psychosis.

Methamphetamine-induced psychosis will usually resolve spontaneously, and first-line treatment should be symptomatic management of agitation and insomnia. Rarely, methamphetamine-induced psychosis can persist for weeks or even months. Anti-psychotic medication may be required if symptoms fail to resolve.

9.6 Management of Acute Health Harms

Cessation of methamphetamine use is likely to be critical in the management of associated acute health harms. For psychiatric harms, such as affective disorders and psychosis, existing evidence-based protocols should be utilised.

9.7 Health Harms from Repeated Use

The chronic adverse health effects of methamphetamine are the same as for other stimulants (see Chapter 6), with particular emphasis on cognitive impairment, mood disorders and psychosis.[51]

Methamphetamine is also associated with injecting-related harms and sexual risk-taking behaviour, and hence the risk of transmission of blood-borne viruses (see Case Study 4, Section 9.8)

Methamphetamine has a high dependence liability and is associated with tolerance and a withdrawal syndrome. Withdrawal from methamphetamine is characterised by psychiatric and physical symptoms similar to those seen with other stimulants.

Acute withdrawal symptoms: Akathisia/restless legs, severe dysphoria, irritability, anxiety, insomnia, fatigue, intense craving, persecutory thinking and suicidal thinking.

Longer-term withdrawal symptoms, which can last weeks to months after discontinuation: Anxiety, mood disturbance, intense craving, impaired social functioning, irritability, insomnia.

9.8 Case 4 Chemsex-Related Sexually Transmitted Infection

Presenting Complaint/History

Andrew is a 24-year-old gay man who has been working as an escort for the last four years. He is HIV negative and takes PREP daily, which he purchases from the internet. Andrew works as an escort three days a week and has approximately eight sexual partners during this period. He always uses condoms and attends for a sexual health screen once a month.

Andrew states that his clients 'expect' him to use drugs with them, and he will often buy drugs and take them with him when meeting a client. He usually buys methamphetamine and GHB, which he uses to enhance his sexual performance.

A week ago, Andrew presented to a local drug service asking for help with his use of methamphetamine, which he felt had become a problem. He described his use as escalating over the last three months, and he was now also using on the days he was not seeing clients, something he had never done previously. Over the preceding three months Andrew had also begun to inject rather than smoke methamphetamine, and although he enjoyed the 'massive high' he acknowledged that when intoxicated through injection he became careless with his health and 'broke' his own rules. He gave examples of sharing needles with other people, forgetting to take PREP for up to a week at a time, engaging in condom-less sex and not attending for regular sexual health screening. Andrew was worried about these changes, which he described as 'very out of character' and said 'the Tina is taking control' ('Tina' and 'crystal' are UK street names for methamphetamine)

Assessment

At assessment, Andrew fulfilled the criteria for dependence on methamphetamine, with clear evidence of tolerance, cravings, withdrawal, difficulty controlling the level of use and continued use despite harmful consequences.

He stated that he wanted to stop using methamphetamine completely but was not sure how he could continue working as an escort without using drugs.

He also agreed to attend an assessment at the local sexual health service.

Andrew told staff that he had not experienced 'sober sex' for more than a decade.

Management

Unfortunately, the sexual health screen showed that Andrew was now HIV and Hepatitis C positive; he also screened positive for chlamydia, syphilis and gonorrhoea. Treatment was commenced for his sexually transmitted infections, including HIV, and a referral was made to the hepatology team.

The drug treatment team met with Andrew weekly and used a relapse prevention approach to support him to achieve abstinence. He continued to experience severe cravings for methamphetamine and was prescribed Naltrexone 50mg daily, with good effect. After several meetings, Andrew accepted that he could not continue to work as an escort without using drugs. He decided that he could only remain abstinent by stopping escorting completely and began to consider other options. With the help of the clinic he began attending a computer course, and at the same time started volunteering twice a week at a local health charity.

Andrew also engaged in psychosexual counselling to discuss his attitude to physical intimacy and how he could begin to consider this without using psychoactive substances.

Key Learning

The use of drugs to facilitate sexual performance and pleasure (chemsex) puts a person at risk of both drug- and sexually related harms, with the disinhibiting effect of drugs such as methamphetamine particularly increasing the risks.

All people who use drugs should be asked about associated sexual behaviours and offered a review at the local sexual health clinic if appropriate.

People who engage in 'chemsex' may find physical intimacy without drugs very difficult. Psychosexual counselling can be helpful for this group.

9.9 Methamphetamine Pro-sexual Effects

Methamphetamine increases sexual drive, decreases fatigue and causes a loss of sexual inhibition. It can delay ejaculation, assist in prolonging intercourse and decrease humoral secretions. Paradoxically, there is also evidence that long-term use can in some cases be associated with decreased sexual functioning.[52]

9.9.1 Chemsex

In some parts of the world, including the UK, there is increasing awareness of the use of stimulant drugs to enhance sexual performance, particularly by a minority of MSM in a pattern of behaviour sometimes called 'chemsex' or 'party and play'. This term is used to describe sex between men that occurs under the influence of drugs which are consumed immediately before and/or during the sexual session. The term 'chemsex' tends to be used to described combined drug use and sexual behaviours within MSM with the goal of sexual enhancement; however, drug use for sexual enhancement can occur in other groups, including heterosexuals.

Drug use for sexual enhancement is associated with high levels of risk relating to both drug harms and sexual behaviours among men who have sex with men[53] as well heterosexuals.[54]

Methamphetamine, mephedrone and GHB/GBL have been particularly identified as drugs used for enhancing sexual performance by increasing sexual arousal and disinhibition. The function of chemsex is often group sexual interaction, with sessions sometimes involving a high number of sexual partners over a short period.

Location-based, social networking applications (e.g. mobile phone apps) have an important role in the procurement of both sexual partners and 'chemsex' drugs. This technology has been described as a facilitator of drug use during sex among MSM and is typically linked with high-risk drug use and sexual behaviours.[56][57]

The types of problems associated with chemsex include high-risk sexual activities and injecting – indeed, for some people injecting appears to have become sexualised – and in particular the sharing of injecting equipment.

However, it is also important to bear in mind that every use of a drug in a sexual context is not necessarily associated with harm,[1] and some have argued that the element of pleasure must not be overlooked in an individual's trajectory of sexualised drug use.[57]

9.10 Management of Health Harms from Repeated Use

9.10.1 Managing the Presentation of 'Chemsex'

The management of people engaging in chemsex will to some extent depend on the clinical presentation and the individual's identified harms and treatment goals. A full assessment of drug-using and sexual behaviours is indicated, including a sexual health screen. Drug treatment staff may require additional training to develop the cultural competence and assessment skills needed to undertake this complex assessment.

Many people engaging in chemsex identify both drug use and sexual behaviours as problematic. Identified goals can vary from abstinence to a desire for some form of improved control over drug use. Specialist drug service will usually need to be involved in developing a treatment plan to change patterns of both drug use and sexual behaviour. Clinical outcomes in this group are poorly researched; however, there are sometimes underlying mental health or psychosexual issues which complicate successful drug treatment. For this reason, in addition to standard evidence-based approaches to drug treatment, psychosexual counselling (e.g. supporting the setting of boundaries and facilitating 'sober' sexual practices) and help in the safe use of social media are often indicated.

Stimulant Drugs: MDMA and Drugs with Similar Effects

10.1 Introduction and Brief Pharmacology

The term 'ecstasy' is generally used to refer to MDMA (3,4-methylenedioxymethamphetamine), although a number of other drugs with similar effects have also been referred to as such.

MDMA is an amphetamine-type stimulant (ATS). It shares some of the features of other ATS, such as amphetamine, but there are also significant differences, including greater hallucinogenic and empathogenic effects. MDMA is structurally similar to both ATS and to mescaline-type hallucinogens.[58]

In contrast to typical stimulants, MDMA has multiple actions at different receptors: it is a releaser and reuptake inhibitor of serotonin, dopamine and noradrenaline, which appears to be linked to its euphoric psychostimulant effect. MDMA is also an agonist at the 5-HT_{2A} receptor, the serotonin receptor responsible for hallucinogenic effects.[59]

10.2 Therapeutic Uses of MDMA

In recent years, there has been an increase in the number of studies examining the role and effectiveness of MDMA as a therapeutic agent, especially in the treatment of mood disturbance and post-traumatic stress disorder.[60] At present, the evidence base has not developed sufficiently to draw any firm conclusions.[61]

10.3 The Fall and Rise of MDMA in the UK

Both the prevalence of use and the strength of MDMA have varied considerably over time in the UK.

MDMA is the third most commonly used illicit substance in the UK, following cannabis and powder cocaine. Although its use has been relatively stable among adults in England and Wales, over the last decade use among the 16–24 age group has fluctuated between 2.9% and 5.4%, with a decline in use between 2010 and 2013, followed by a subsequent increase.[62]

This variation in the prevalence of MDMA use has coincided with fluctuations in the availability, quality and strength of MDMA on drug markets. A worldwide shortage of MDMA in the late 2000s probably accounted for the low purity of MDMA in the UK during this period.[63] This has been associated in part with a shortage of the precursor safrole in 2008 (3,4methylenedioxyallybenzene, a liquid extracted from sassafras plants) and later PMK (piperonyl methyl ketone, itself derived from safrole).

It has been argued that this dip in the quality of MDMA may have helped drive the emergence of mephedrone as a club drug.[64] It has been suggested that the increased use of NPS (and mephedrone in particular) was a result of the reduced availability of 'normal' strength MDMA.[69]

This situation has now reversed, with increased availability of high-purity MDMA and a consequent rise in the numbers of people between the ages of 16–24 in particular using the drug. Following a decade of decreasing MDMA/ ecstasy use, the estimated consumption of this drug has risen in several European countries.[65][66][38] A new MDMA precursor called PMK-glycidate became available around 2010, revitalising MDMA production. PMK-glycidate is not derived from safrole and is therefore not vulnerable to natural shortages.[67]

Indeed, in the mid-2000s in Europe, the mean dose of MDMA was estimated to be 50–80mg. By 2016, the mean dose reported in Europe was approximately 125 mg, and batches of very high potency tablets (e.g. containing up to 340 mg) have been identified.[73] The majority of MDMA available in the UK is thought to originate in the Netherlands, where the proportion of MDMA manufactured containing more than 140 mg has risen from 3% in 2009 to 53% in 2015. In 2016, 75% of MDMA powder at user-level in the UK was more than 140 mg per tablet.[68]

Data on deaths where MDMA was detected at post-mortem reflect this fluctuation (Figure 10.1). There was a sharp drop in the number of MDMA-related deaths in 2009, but this has now reverted to (and even exceeded) the previous higher levels. MDMA was mentioned in 56 cases in 2017 and 92 cases in 2018, in comparison to 8 in 2010 and 13 in 2011.[13]

A number of NPS have been developed with effects similar to those of MDMA. These substances have in some cases been marketed and sold as new alternatives to MDMA. In other cases, the NPS are deliberately mis-sold as MDMA to unsuspecting customers, sometimes leading to severe adverse effects.

10.4 Substitution of MDMA with Other Drugs

Paramethoxyamphetamine (PMA) and paramethoxymethamphetamine (PMMA) are some of the substances which have been substituted for

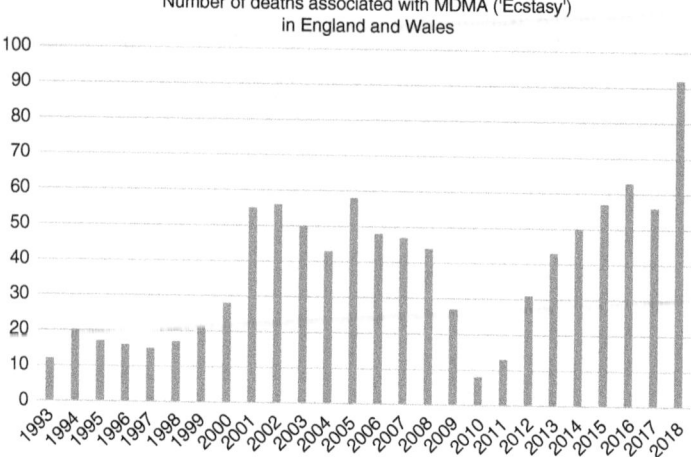

Figure 10.1 Number of deaths per year where MDMA was implicated (England and Wales)[13]

MDMA, or added to products that also contain MDMA or other substances. They are potent noradrenaline and serotonin transporter inhibitors and also releasers of these monoamines. As a consequence they have a high potential to cause life-threatening toxicity and have been associated with severe harms and deaths.[69]

People who use PMA and PMMA unknowingly risk overdosing as these substances have a slow onset of ecstasy-like effects in comparison to MDMA. This can lead to users to believe that they have taken weaker ecstasy, resulting in consumption of further doses and subsequent toxicity. In addition, compared with MDMA, PMA and PMMA appear to have a higher potential to cause life-threatening hyperthermia.[70]

N-ethyl pentylone and its analogues are also mis-sold as MDMA. Initially they have quite similar psychoactive effects to MDMA; however, the empathogenic effects of pentylone are not so pronounced and the euphoria fades more quickly, often leading to re-dosing. [79]

10.5 Modes of Use

MDMA is available in a number of forms, most commonly as powder/crystals or as tablets and capsules.

MDMA is absorbed rapidly. It typically takes 20–60 minutes for the psychoactive effect to be experienced, reaching peak effects between 60 and 90 minutes, and lasting up to 5 hours. The half-life of a dose of 100 mg is around 8–9 hours.[71]

10.6 Desired Effects by User

MDMA produces stimulant effects, such as increased energy and euphoria, broadly similar to those of other amphetamine-type substances. In addition, it also produces characteristic alterations of mood and perception, particularly increased empathy, emotional well-being, sociability (pro-social effects) and sensuality. The terms 'entactogens' or 'empathogens' have been used to describe these drug effects.[72]

10.7 Acute Health Harms

The general acute and chronic harms of MDMA are similar to those of other stimulants and are discussed in Chapter 6.

Hospital presentations associated with the use of MDMA and other similar substances fall into a number of overlapping clinical categories listed below. The clinical presentation may be further complicated by impurities or other substances mixed into the preparation, as well as concomitant drug and alcohol use. [73]

10.7.1 Acute physical presentations

Hyperthermia and serotonin syndrome are two life-threatening effects of MDMA intoxication. These are discussed in more detail in Case Study 5 (Section 10.9).

Dilutional hyponatraemia and hyponatraemic encephalopathy can be the result of excessive fluid intake by the individual. Hyponatraemia seems to be particularly a cause of MDMA-related fatalities in women.[74]

Other physiological harms include cardiac events, liver failure and pneumomediastinum. MDMA produces cardiovascular effects broadly similar to those of other amphetamine-type substances and cocaine.

10.7.2 Acute Psychiatric Presentations

Marked anxiety is a common presentation among people who have used MDMA and are seeking medical help. Despite its relatively high prevalence of use, evidence linking MDMA to psychosis is limited.[75]

10.8 Management of Acute Health Harms

The management of acute adverse effects of MDMA should follow the same protocols as for other stimulant drugs.

10.8.1 Serotonin Syndrome

MDMA can cause severe serotonin poisoning (known as serotonin syndrome) and has sympathomimetic effects. For more information on presentation and clinical management, see Chapter 6.

10.8.2 Management of Hyperthermia and Hyperpyrexia

Hyperthermia and hyperpyrexia are life-threatening adverse reactions to MDMA and have been associated with death.[76]

- Most cases will have self-limiting symptoms that require minimal intervention, including correcting dehydration and allowing rest.
- For a minority of cases, however, hyperthermia or hyperpyrexia will be severe and will not resolve spontaneously with rest in a cooler environment.

A range of severe complications are associated with significant hyperthermia, including sudden collapse, cardiac arrest, disseminated intravascular coagulation, protracted seizures, multiple organ failure, metabolic acidosis, neuromuscular hyperactivity, rhabdomyolysis and death.[29]

TOXBASE® suggests that mild to moderate hyperthermia may respond to conventional cooling measures such as mist and fan techniques, ice packs and external cooling devices.

Patients presenting with rising body temperatures that exceed 38°C, require urgent cooling measures with regular monitoring of core temperature. Cooling measures include:

- Ice-baths
- Internal/invasive measures: cold fluid lavage (gastric, bladder, peritoneal), intravascular cooling techniques
- Sedation should be employed where it can be safely performed.

Severe hyperthermia carries a high mortality rate and rapid intervention is recommended. TOXBASE® suggests that rapid sequence intubation with paralysis is usually warranted when the temperature is rising rapidly and is not controlled by the above measures. They also recommend ongoing neuromuscular paralysis and sedation with benzodiazepines in addition to cooling measures.

Some have suggested that dantrolene may be considered if there is muscular hyperactivity and hyperthermia persists; however, a 2011 evaluation of options in MDMA-induced hyperthermia recommended against the use dantrolene or other antipyretic medication.[77]

10.8.3 Management of Hyponatraemia and Fluid Overload

MDMA is typically used at dance venues to increase energy and enhance the experience of the music and light show. Prolonged exertion and sweating can result in reduced blood sodium levels. When this is combined with the consumption of excessive quantities of low-electrolyte fluids such as beer and water, hyponataemia can occur and can be severe.

The symptoms of dilutional hyponatraemia result mostly from the progression of cerebral swelling. Initial headache, vomiting and disturbed mental state are followed by drowsiness, disorientation, muteness and seizures, progressing to coma, hypoxia and death, often due to tentorial herniation.[78]

Patients with hyponatraemia will require fluid restriction, so it is dangerous to give people with MDMA-related hyperthermia hypotonic fluids or normal saline prior to proper assessment.[79] It has been recommended that in all patients with hyponatraemia, free water intake from all sources should be restricted to less than 1–1.5 l per 24 hours and water restriction will gradually increase the serum sodium concentration. It is argued that in patients with mild symptoms, the rate of urinary solute excretion can be increased by a high-salt, high-protein diet or supplementation with urea or salt tablets, but salt therapy is generally contraindicated in patients with hypertension and oedema. Symptomatic or severe hyponatraemia generally requires hospitalisation for observation, careful monitoring of fluid balance and body weight, and frequent measurements of plasma sodium concentrations. It is also suggested that laboratory tests should include plasma osmolality, urine osmolality and urine sodium. Additional tests of thyroid and adrenal function may also be necessary.[80]

10.9 Case 5 MDMA-Induced Serotonin Syndrome

Presenting Complaint/History

Sally is a 19-year-old university student studying Business. She enjoys university and is popular and sociable, attending events with friends most weekends. This weekend, Sally is going clubbing with four friends and they meet at a local pub first. They each drink 6 standard alcohol units before arriving at a club around midnight. One of Sally's friends, with the agreement of everyone, has bought some tablets of MDMA, which she smuggles past security.

Once inside, all five friends take one tablet of MDMA. Sally has previously taken MDMA on around 20 occasions and experiences the familiar euphoria and energy rush about 20 minutes after ingestion. An hour later, Sally takes a second tablet as she feels the effects of the first tablet wearing off. The second tablet works much faster and the effects feel stronger. Sally goes back to the dance floor with her friends but soon begins to feel overheated and nauseous. She tells one of her friends that she feels unwell and they take her to sit down. Sally becomes increasingly distressed and tells her friend that her heart is racing and that she feels dizzy. She is sweating and begins to shiver. Not knowing what to do, her friend takes Sally out of the club for some fresh air. Sally is now very agitated and has become confused, not knowing where she is or recognising her friend. An ambulance is called and Sally is taken to hospital. On the way to the hospital, the paramedics secure IV access, check Sally's blood sugar, which is within normal range, and administer paracetamol.

Assessment

On arrival at the Emergency Department, Sally is tachycardic, hypertensive, hyperthermic and diaphoretic. There is evidence of increased muscle tone, particularly pronounced in her legs, with marked hyperreflexia and clonus. She is significantly confused, with disorientation in time, person and place.

Bloods revealed a raised creatinine kinase and a slightly raised lactate. Serum sodium is within normal range.

A diagnosis of serotonin syndrome is made.

Management

Management involves supportive treatment, including benzodiazepines for agitation and IV fluids. Rapid cooling is initiated and the situation is discussed with ITU. Consideration is given to dantrolene, intubation and multi-organ support.

Key Learning

Serotonin syndrome is a rare but potentially life-threatening condition resulting from excess serotonergic agonism.

Symptoms can range from mild to severe and include a classical triad of

- neuromuscular abnormalities (hyperreflexia, peripheral hypertonicity)
- autonomic hyperactivity (tachycardia, hyperpyrexia)
- mental state changes (agitated delirium)

Serotonin syndrome can be life threatening and requires urgent medical assessment and intervention. See Chapter 6.

10.10   Health Harms from Repeated Use

Like other ATS, the period following MDMA use can be followed by an initial dysphoric 'crash'. In regular users, this may be followed by an extended 'withdrawal' phase, marked by anhedonia and anergia.[81] MDMA users sometimes refer to 'mid-week blues' to describe symptoms that typically appear 3–5 days after last use of MDMA. Novice users may suffer fatigue, depressed mood and decreased appetite in the days after use. Regular use appears to be linked to an increase in intensity and incidence of these symptoms as well as other symptoms, such as nightmares and difficulty with memory and concentration.[82]

It has been suggested that many of these effects are associated with depletion of serotonin.[35] For people vulnerable to depressive disorder, these symptoms could be exacerbated.[83]

MDMA has some dependence potential, but this is relatively weak in comparison with other stimulants. Use is often self-limiting and focused around recreational activities and it has been suggested that the low dependence potential is partially linked to the relatively long period of recovery after one dose.[84]

Nonetheless, studies have shown that people who use MDMA may fulfil dependence criteria, develop problematic chronic use patterns, have concerns about their use, find it difficult abstain and sometimes seek treatment.[85]

It has been argued that although the physiological basis of MDMA dependence is relatively weak in comparison with some other ATS, other behavioural and psychological factors will contribute to dependence on MDMA.[86]

10.11 Management of Health Harms from Repeated Use

The management of the harmful or dependent use of MDMA is primarily psycho-social and similar to that provided to people with the harmful or dependent use of other stimulants.

Typically, people with harmful or dependent use of MDMA will also be poly-drug users, and assessment and interventions should address all drug and alcohol use, as well as any co-existing mental health problems.

Stimulant Drugs: Synthetic Cathinones

11.1 Introduction

Synthetic cathinones are also ATS and have some effects that are broadly similar to both methamphetamines and MDMA.

Synthetic cathinones are one of the largest groups of NPS detected globally, with 148 synthetic cathinones reported to the UNODC by the end of 2017.[1] The European Drug Report 2019 stated that in Europe, synthetic cathinones are the second largest group of new substances monitored by the EMCDDA, with 130 detected in total.[6]

The most common synthetic cathinone detected globally, as well as in the UK, is mephedrone. Other commonly detected synthetic cathinones include:

Methylenedioxypyrovalerone (MDPV)

Methylone (3,4-methylenedioxy-N-methcathinone)

Naphyrone (naphthylpyrovalerone)

α-Pyrrolidinopentiophenone (alpha-PVP)

4-methyl-N-ethylcathinone (4-MEC)

4'-Methyl-α-pyrrolidinopropiophenone (4-MePPP)

3',4'-Methylenedioxy-α-pyrrolidinohexiophenone (MDPHP)

Synthetic cathinone use shows considerable geographical variation. For example, mephedrone has been reported in the UK, alpha-PVP in Finland, pentedrone in Hungary and 3-MMC in Slovenia, while MDPV has often been associated with adverse health effects in the USA.[87]

The prevalence of cathinone use appears to be markedly dynamic, with particular substances gaining then losing popularity, often over a few months. As with other NPS, 'second generation' substances have been developed from earlier compounds, and may be associated with high toxicity.

11.2 Brief Pharmacology

Cathinones stimulate the release of and inhibit the reuptake of adrenaline, noradrenaline and serotonin.[88]

Different synthetic cathinones have considerable variation in structure and psychopharmacology, leading to differing potency and toxicity.[87]

Pharmacological Differences Between Synthetic Cathinones

There are differences in the mechanisms of action of the various synthetic cathinones. For example, mephedrone acts primarily by releasing dopamine, whereas MDPV is a dopamine reuptake inhibitor. Mephedrone and MDPV therefore behave through different mechanisms, with mephedrone's action being similar to drugs such as methamphetamine (pre-synaptic dopamine releaser), while MDPV's action is similar to cocaine (dopamine reuptake inhibitor).[89]

11.3 Modes of Use

11.3.1 Mephedrone

Mephedrone was one of the first commonly used NPS in the UK and globally. It is an amphetamine-type analogue structurally related to amphetamine, methamphetamine and MDMA.

Mephedrone and other synthetic cathinones are typically used orally, often wrapped in paper and swallowed.[90] They can also be snorted or injected.

The onset of the desired effects of mephedrone is linked to the route of administration: a few minutes following snorting or intravenous injection and 15–45 minutes following oral ingestion.

The duration of the effects is linked to mode of use. The effects last up to 2–3 hours following oral use, a shorter duration when ingested through nasal insufflation, but only 15–30 minutes following intravenous use. The relatively short duration of effect of mephedrone is associated with frequent repeated dosing during a single session.[91] [106]

11.3.2 MDPV

MDPV is typically supplied as a white or white–tan coloured powder; there are also reports of tablet, capsule and liquid forms. MDPV is soluble in water and the powder can be dissolved for oral use or intravenous and subcutaneous injection.

MDPV has been detected in paper blotters, and there have been reports of MDPV being sprayed onto vegetable material intended for smoking. Information from user websites suggests that rectal administration may also be a potential route. The most common routes of administration for MDPV are nasal (insufflation/ sniffing) and oral (swallowing).

The onset of desired effects is typically seen within 5–30 minutes, with desired effects lasting 2–7 hours for the common routes of administration (oral and nasal).

Repeated dosing of MDPV has also been noted.[91]

11.4 Desired Effects by User

Commonly reported desired effects of synthetic cathinones include:[92] [93] [94]

- Mood enhancement – including euphoria
- Energy enhancement – reduced need for sleep
- Cognitive enhancement – improved concentration
- Social enhancement – increased sociability and confidence, increased empathy
- Sexual enhancement – heightened sensuality, disinhibition, prolonged sexual performance

11.5 Acute Health Harms

Acute adverse health effects of synthetic cathinones include fatigue, persistent negative mood, suicidal thoughts, anxiety, panic attacks, excited delirium, bouts of violent aggression towards self and others, and combativeness that resemble a severe psychotic episode.[94] [95]

The toxicity of synthetic cathinones is generally similar to that of amphetamines. Some synthetic cathinones also have negative effects that are similar to those of cocaine or MDMA.

Synthetic cathinones produce sympathomimetic clinical effects consistent with stimulant intoxication. They may be associated with greater risk of neurotoxicity in comparison to traditional stimulants. [96] [97] [98]

Cardiac, psychiatric and neurological symptoms are the most commonly reported effects that require medical care.[99] The use of synthetic cathinones has been associated with hyperthermia, similar to that linked to MDMA use.[100] Serotonin syndrome may also occur, especially when the user has been exposed to two or more serotonergic drugs or when regularly consuming them.

11.6 Management of Acute Health Harms

It has been argued that, given the similarities with cocaine and amphetamine, management strategies similar to those recommended for intoxication with those drugs might be useful.[101] Symptom-directed supportive care for acute stimulant intoxication may include the management of agitation, convulsions, metabolic acidosis, hypertension, hypotension and rhabdomyolysis. The management of serotonin syndrome may also be indicated. The literature contains reports of the use of antipsychotics, but these should be used cautiously with synthetic cathinone intoxication as they may increase seizure activity.[102]

11.7 Health Harms from Repeated Use

Prolonged use of cathinones can lead to similar consequences as seen with other stimulant drugs, including dependence and associated mental health problems.

11.7.1 Dependence on Cathinones

- There is increasing evidence that synthetic cathinones have a misuse liability, are linked to a strong and repeated compulsion to use and have a dependence potential.[10]
- Synthetic cathinones have a higher risk of dependence than MDMA.[103] Some studies suggest that the dependence potential for MDPV is greater than for methamphetamine, but this is not seen in all studies.[104]
- People who use synthetic cathinones frequently develop tolerance.[105] [106]
- Dependence symptoms have been described as similar to those generally observed in cocaine or amphetamines misuse, including loss of control, craving and tolerance.[107]
- A withdrawal syndrome, similar to that associated with other stimulants, has been described in heavier users. Symptoms include tiredness, insomnia, impaired concentration, irritability, nasal congestion, tremor, shivers, increased or decreased temperature, palpitations, headache, depression, anxiety and paranoia.[108]

11.7.2 Injecting

The intravenous injecting of synthetic cathinones may be associated with more severe symptomatology and greater dependence liability.

The injection of synthetic cathinones has been associated with a range of high-risk behaviours and harms.[109]

Injectors also report intense burning sensations at injection sites, limb abscesses and vein damage. These result from drug toxicity, crystallisation of the drug when diluted and syringe flushing practices. They also report multi-drug and serial drug injecting. The limited research describing this practice strongly suggests its potential for health harms. Intravenous users of mephedrone report parasitosis (leading to scratching and gouging of the skin of the face, necks and arms in particular), severe insomnia, and persecutory and suicidal thinking, especially after prolonged use.[99]

11.8 Case 6 Mephedrone Injecting

Presenting Complaint/History

Terry is a 27-year-old man who has been street homeless for more than a year. He occasionally meets an outreach worker but otherwise has no contact with health services. Terry has used a number of drugs in the past, most notably heroin. He injected heroin in his arms for four years, but stopped using while serving a three-month custodial sentence. Since release, his main drug has been alcohol and he consumes around 10 standard alcohol units daily.

Six months ago Terry was introduced to mephedrone by someone on the street. He was told the 'best' way to use it was by injection, and Terry began injecting once more. He found it difficult to successfully inject into the veins in his arms and so started injecting into his hands, feet and groin (femoral vein). Terry noticed that mephedrone caused more damage to his veins than the heroin he was used to and that he also needed to inject more frequently. He needed to attend the Emergency Room on several occasions as he had developed abscesses that did not heal.

Terry gradually increased the frequency of mephedrone injecting and now will often inject between six and ten times a day – much more frequently than when he used to inject heroin. He explains to the outreach worker that he craves another injection soon after the last one is finished.

Recently, Terry told his outreach worker that an injection in his groin had 'gone wrong': he experienced a sharp pain in his groin and 'a lot of blood'. Although the bleeding had stopped, Terry found it difficult to walk, as every step caused excruciating pain in his groin. The outreach worker strongly suggested that Terry attend the Emergency Room and offered to accompany him, but Terry said he would rather 'wait a bit' to see if it improved.

Ten days later and still unable to walk, Terry went to the Emergency Room.

Assessment
At assessment, there is a large haematoma in the left inguinal region, indicating that the patient may have accidentally injected into his femoral artery. The area also appears to be infected and the patient is pyrexial with a raised white cell count. Further examination also suggests that the femoral nerve may also be damaged, although it is unclear if this is the result of direct trauma from the needle or secondary to localised infection.

Management
Terry is offered admission and intravenous antibiotics. Due to his poor venous access, a central line is considered. Unfortunately, while staff are arranging the bed, Terry decides he does not want medical treatment and leaves. He returns to injecting mephedrone that evening. A week later, his outreach worker finds him sleeping in a doorway. Terry explains that he used a friend's antibiotics and is feeling much better. He is still experiencing difficulty walking but thinks it is improving. His outreach worker again offers to take him to hospital for a checkup but Terry declines.

Key Learning
Injecting of cathinones such as mephedrone can lead to compulsive and frequent dosing.

The increased frequency of injecting and the drug effects combine to cause higher rates of complications, including abscesses.

Homeless people who use drugs can be difficult to engage in mainstream health services but benefit from specialised, flexible treatment approaches.

11.9   Management of Harms from Repeated Use

Mephedrone Dependence

For the management of mephedrone dependence, use existing protocols for stimulant dependence (see Chapter 6).

Chapter

12

Depressant Drugs: Introduction

In this part, we will examine emerging drugs with primarily depressant effects on the central nervous system. Although the number of these is relatively small in comparison to emerging stimulants and synthetic cannabinoids, the number of new depressant drugs is growing.

Different classes of depressant drugs work in different ways, with common mechanisms being agonism of opioid or GABA receptor systems. Depressants may also inhibit excitatory glutamatergic or catecholaminergic activity (dopamine, noradrenaline, and epinephrine). However, some depressant drugs, such as GHB/GBL, at low doses also release noradrenaline, causing mild stimulant effects when small amounts are consumed.

In this part we will look at GHB, new synthetic opioids and new benzodiazepines. In addition, and because of their primarily depressant effects, we have also included dissociative drugs, such as ketamine.

This part will focus on the misuse of these drugs and their use in recreational settings. It will not cover their legitimate medicinal use in clinical settings.

Depressant Drugs: Gamma-Hydroxybutyrate (GHB) and Gamma-Butyrolactone (GBL)

13.1 Introduction and Brief Pharmacology

Although use of GHB and GBL is relatively limited in most countries, they have high health costs compared with other drugs because of their intrinsic toxicity, overdose risk, high dependence liability and potentially life-threatening withdrawal syndrome.

Gamma-hydroxybutyrate (GHB) and its precursor gamma-butyrolactone (GBL) are central nervous system (CNS) depressants. GHB is both a metabolite and a precursor of gamma-aminobutyric acid (GABA)[110] and acts on both GABA-B and at their own so-called GHB receptors. GHB/GBL also release noradrenaline and therefore produce, at low doses, euphoric effects similar to those of stimulants.[111] The effects of GHB usually occur 15–20 minutes after ingestion, with peak effects at 30–60 minutes after use. Effects can last for up to 3–4 hours. GHB is undetectable in urine after approximately 12 hours.[112]

GBL is non-enzymatically converted in the body into GHB. GBL is absorbed more rapidly than GHB and potentially has a faster onset of action. Its duration of action may also be longer.[113]

Less commonly consumed, but related substances include Gamma-hydroxyvaleric acid (GHV), which is available for sale on the internet and marketed as a food supplement and replacement for GHB.[114] GHV is a 4-methyl-substituted analogue of GHB and a direct GABA receptor agonist. Gamma-valerolactone (GVL) is a precursor of GHV. Larger doses of GHV may be needed to produce GHB-like effects and therefore people may use large quantities to produce these effects, leading to the risk of overdose.[114]

13.2 Modes of Use

GHB/GBL are most commonly sold as clear liquids and are typically consumed diluted in a non-alcoholic beverage. Other preparations are also available, including powder.

13.3   Desired Effects by User

The desired effects of GHB/GBL include euphoria, relaxation and sedation. GHB/GBL are sometimes used to assist with insomnia. The substances also have pro-sexual and smooth muscle relaxant effects which likely explains their use for 'chemsex', often in combination with stimulant drugs such as methamphetamine. This pattern of use is most commonly observed in men who have sex with men.

13.4   Acute Health Harms

GHB/GBL are associated with severe acute adverse health effects resulting from:

- Acute toxicity and overdose
- Severe withdrawal syndrome in dependent individuals

GHB/GBL can readily cross both the placenta and the blood–brain barrier, and can lead to profound CNS and respiratory depression and death.[111] The symptoms of acute toxicity vary depending on dose, ranging from drowsiness to profound coma.

GHB/GBL has a steep dose–response curve. Even a small increase in dose, or the use of another CNS depressant, can cause serious toxic effects, such as impaired consciousness and coma. Effects can be brought on by imprecise dosing and are potentiated by co-ingestion of other CNS depressants such as alcohol, benzodiazepines, antipsychotics and some illicit drugs.[115]

13.4.1   Acute Toxicity

Overdoses with loss of consciousness are commonly reported by GHB/GBL users.[116] The usual clinical course involves a rapid onset of drowsiness leading to loss of consciousness. Recovery is typically rapid and uneventful. CNS depression usually persists for 1–3 hours, with patients typically making a full recovery within 4–8 hours.[117] GHB/GBL have the unusual property that people can progress from deep coma to wakefulness, and vice versa, in a few minutes.

TOXBASE® (the poisons information database of the National Poisons Information Service (NPIS)), summarises the acute effects of GHB/GBL toxicity as follows:[118]

- **Mild/moderate** effects include nausea, hypersalivation, vomiting, diarrhoea, drowsiness, headache, ataxia, dizziness, confusion, amnesia, urinary incontinence, tremor, myoclonus, hypotonia, agitation, euphoria and hypothermia.

- **In severe cases** there may be bradycardia, ECG abnormalities (including U waves, inverted P waves, QRS and QT prolongation, AV block and atrial fibrillation), hypotension (or, rarely, hypertension after intravenous use), and respiratory depression leading to respiratory arrest, rhabdomyolysis, convulsions and coma. Metabolic acidosis has been reported.

Laboratory abnormalities may include hypernatraemia, hypokalaemia and hyperglycaemia.

In GHB/GBL-dependent people, rapid improvement from acute toxicity may be followed by deterioration as withdrawal symptoms develop. It has been recommended that a vital part of discharge instructions to patients, friends and carers is to inform them about the potential for withdrawal symptoms occurring after discharge[119] and the importance of seeking immediate medical help if these develop.

13.4.2 Withdrawal Syndrome

GHB/GBL withdrawal syndrome is only seen in those who are dependent. Dependent users will typically be using daily, and often multiple times a day. Withdrawal syndrome, as with withdrawal from other psychoactive substances, usually occurs on reduction or cessation of the drug. Withdrawal symptoms typically manifest quickly (in under an hour), but have been reported up to 24–48 hours after the last dose.

There are wide differences between individuals in the severity of the withdrawal symptoms they experience and their response to clinical interventions, independent of the severity of dependence. GHB/GBL withdrawal can be life threatening and must be treated as a medical emergency, particularly if the patient is already in severe withdrawal at the time of presentation.

The symptoms of GHB/GBL withdrawal usually include insomnia, tremor, nausea and vomiting, anxiety, agitation, disorientation, confusion, depression, nystagmus, diarrhoea, tachypnoea, dyspnoea, tachycardia, hypertension and abdominal pain. Hallucinations (auditory and visual), convulsions and/or myoclonic jerks may develop. There are also reports of pyrexia, muscle rigidity, rhabdomyolysis, acute renal failure and hypo- or hyperkalaemia.[118]

The symptoms of GHB/GBL withdrawal syndrome can be self-limiting in some people, but others can experience more severe withdrawal that can progress to delirium.[120]

Abrupt decrease or discontinuation of heavy GHB use may result in a severe and life-threatening withdrawal syndrome characterised by autonomic instability, delirium and aggression.[121]

GHB/GBL withdrawal syndrome can appear clinically similar to withdrawal from other psychoactive drugs, including opioids, benzodiazepines and alcohol. Assessment of all psychoactive drug use is therefore essential.

The clinical picture of GHB/GBL withdrawal is similar to the alcohol withdrawal syndrome; however, neuropsychiatric features may be more prominent. Symptoms may also be more prolonged (up to 2 weeks, occasionally longer) and are typically more resistant to benzodiazepines.[118]

GHB/GBL withdrawal can also have similarities to other clinical presentations, such as hypoglycaemia or to acute sympathomimetic drug toxicity, typically associated with stimulant use.

13.5 Case 7 Acute GHB Withdrawal

Presenting Complaint/History

John is a 29-year-old man living with his boyfriend, Alan. John is an IT consultant and runs his own company. The firm has been very successful and John enjoys the work but finds it very stressful. John and Alan use drugs around once a month to facilitate physical intimacy. They usually use methamphetamine by smoking and GHB diluted in a drink. The couple do not use drugs in other settings, neither drink alcohol at all and they both regularly attend the gym to keep fit.

Six months ago, John took on a new, large contract. He knew it would be a significant amount of work, but felt that it was a good step for his company to undertake a larger-than-usual project. Within a month, John felt overwhelmed by the complexity of the work and the frequent requests of the demanding clients. He worked even longer hours, returning home each night exhausted and already worrying about the next day's tasks. He developed insomnia, often waking several times a night worried about having miscalculated something at work. After a few weeks, he started taking zopiclone, which he had bought online, but found this unhelpful. A friend suggested that he tried a 'tiny bit of G' and so John experimented with taking 0.5ml of GHB before he went to bed. To his surprise, he found this completely resolved his insomnia. He slept without interruption and woke each morning feeling refreshed. After one week of excellent sleep, John tried sleeping without the GHB but found his insomnia returned immediately. He returned to using GHB and again slept well.

Over the next few weeks John used GHB most nights. Each time he tried to stop he could not sleep and decided he would allow himself to take GHB nightly until the project was complete, which was estimated to be in a few weeks' time. He noticed that the quantity of GHB he needed to achieve a full night's sleep was slowly increasing, but made a mental note not to allow the dose to increase beyond 1.5mls per night.

At the end of the month, the project was not complete and was running about a month late. John encouraged his team to make a final push to finish the contract and increased his own hours further, working every weekend. His GHB use was now at 1.5mls per night. John had started to feel restless, sweaty and agitated during the day, with marked cravings for GHB. He recognised that he may be becoming dependent on GHB but felt he had no choice but to continue using it until the project was complete. He began to take 0.5 ml in the morning before work, but this quickly escalated to 0.5mls twice during the day and 2mls at night. Alan expressed concern about John becoming dependent, but John reassured him that it was only for another few weeks and then he would stop. Unfortunately the project needed to be extended once again as the clients were not completely happy with the work. John's GHB use now escalated rapidly to 1.5mls every three to four hours with 3mls at night before bed. Despite this, John experienced withdrawals during the night and had to take an extra 1.5mls around 3am to stop the sweating and agitation he was experiencing. In total, John was consuming around 15mls of GHB daily.

Finally, the project was concluded and the clients were happy with the result. John knew that he now had to tackle his GHB dependence and tried several times to stop but could not tolerate the severity of the withdrawals. On one occasion John became sweaty, distressed and confused. Alarmed, Alan took him to the Emergency Room where he was given diazepam, but John decided to return home to take more GHB before the psychiatric liaison team arrived. After searching the internet, he found a local drug service that specialised in GHB.

Assessment

John made an appointment and went to an initial assessment with the hope that they could help him stop using GHB. At the drug service, John began to experience GHB withdrawals towards the end of the assessment and needed to leave early to re-dose with GHB. He returned the next day to complete the assessment. He identified his goal as complete abstinence from GHB. A urinary drug screen was negative for all drugs (most standard urine tests do not detect GHB). Physical examination was unremarkable and there were no co-existing mental health problems detected.

A diagnosis of GHB dependence was made, with a plan to undertake an elective, medically assisted detoxification.

Management

Over the next few meetings at the clinic, John worked with staff to develop a post-detoxification plan, including identification of triggering situations, managing cravings and an emergency plan should he begin to relapse. Alan also attended some of these meeting to help support John.

The detoxification was conducted at the clinic using a combination of diazepam and baclofen. The Clinical Institute Withdrawal Assessment for alcohol (CIWA) was used in the absence of a specific validated GHB withdrawal scale. Alan attended with John and took him home each day with a clear plan of what to do if there were any problems. After 4 days, John was making good progress, and the diazepam was slowly tapered down over the following week. Baclofen was continued for a further two weeks as John found this medication very helpful at reducing his cravings.

A month later, John had not consumed any GHB. He continued to attend the clinic on a weekly basis for relapse prevention work and also employed more staff at his company to reduce his workload, something he identified as a significant future trigger. John and Alan worked with the clinic's psychosexual therapist to help them enjoy physical intimacy without the need for psychoactive substances.

Key Learning
GHB dependence can develop after a few weeks of heavy use, with marked withdrawal symptoms.

GHB withdrawals can be severe and even life threatening

Careful planning is needed for medically assisted GHB withdrawals, including post-detoxification planning.

Although elective, medically assisted GHB withdrawals can be undertaken in the community, careful consideration needs to be given to the potential risks of this approach. Unless the team is experienced in managing GHB withdrawals and the level of dependence is low, then an inpatient setting is recommended.

13.6   Management of Acute Health Harms

13.6.1   Management of Acute Intoxication
Acute intoxication with GHB/GBL is managed with supportive care. No antidote is available. Most patients will respond quickly and make a full recovery. Occasionally, management in an intensive care setting is indicated; however, prognosis is still usually good.

13.6.2   Management of Withdrawal Syndrome

Planned Medically Assisted Withdrawal
It is strongly recommended that people dependent on GHB/GBL who wish to stop should seek a medically assisted detoxification. Self-detoxification without medical supervision should be avoided. Detoxification from GHB/GBL can be dangerous, as withdrawal symptoms can be severe and potentially life threatening.

Treatment Setting: Inpatient or Outpatient?
There are no national or international criteria for determining the most appropriate setting for an elective GHB/GBL detoxification. In the absence of clear guidance it is suggested that the setting (community or inpatient) be determined by considering the following patient and service factors:

Patient Factors Suggesting an Inpatient Detoxification

- Severe dependence (>32mls/day or dosing of every 2 hours or less)
- Dosing through the night (unable to sleep more than 4 hours without dosing)
- Significant co-existing physical or psychiatric comorbidity
- Co-existing harmful or dependent benzodiazepine use
- Previous severe GHB/GBL withdrawals
- Previous failed community-based medically assisted detoxification
- Absence of support system to bring the patient to and from appointments and stay with the patient outside of clinic hours

Service Factors Suggesting an Inpatient Detoxification

- Limited clinical staff competence and experience in GHB/GBL detoxification
- Lack of rapidly accessible acute medical support such as intensive care facilities (e.g. likely to be lengthy time period to transfer patient to hospital if needed).

A bio-psychosocial intervention is recommended including the following.

Pharmacological Interventions

The research evidence informing medically assisted elective detoxification from GHB/GBL is limited, but a small number of studies and some case reports have described successful elective, medically assisted detoxification regimens.[122]

Overall, pharmacological interventions described include:

Benzodiazepines:

- To date, a reducing benzodiazepine regimen has been the most commonly described intervention. The use of high doses of benzodiazepines has been described. In the UK at the time of writing, the National Poisons Information Service TOXBASE® states that high doses may be required in severe cases or when treatment is delayed (e.g. in excess of 100 mg of diazepam per 24 hours in divided doses of 10–20 mg at 2–4-hourly intervals).

  Some patients fail to respond to benzodiazepines, even at high doses. In these cases interventions such as general anaesthesia and admission to an intensive care setting may be indicated.

Baclofen:

- The use of baclofen as an adjunct to benzodiazepines has been described, as it is possible that it may reduce the severity of withdrawal symptoms through its activity on the GABA system. TOXBASE® supports the use of baclofen as an adjunct.

· The pre-loading of the patient with baclofen two days before the start of elective detoxification has been described (e.g. 10 mg three times a day), although there is currently limited research evidence to support this approach.[123]

· There is also limited evidence suggesting that patients receiving baclofen after detoxification showed reduced relapse rates compared with patients receiving treatment as usual.[124]

Pharmaceutical GHB:

• There is some evidence supporting the use of pharmaceutical GHB as a safe alternative to benzodiazepine in elective GHB detoxification.[125] [126]

Other:

• There are some reports of patients responding to barbiturate medication in benzodiazepine refractory cases.

The assessment of the patient before the start of an elective detoxification should include other co-occurring drug use, particularly benzodiazepines and alcohol. A urine test to detect any other drug use is essential.

Existing mental health problems, relevant physical health issues (such as a history of seizures) and medication regimens should be carefully considered.

Psycho-Social Interventions

It appears that relapse rates after GHB/GBL detoxification can be as high as 60% within 3 months of detoxification.[124]

There is a large body of evidence on drug treatment and recovery for drug use in general suggesting that psycho-social interventions are an important element of elective detoxification and are linked to treatment success, sustained changes in drug use and abstinence. Although little research has been conducted directly relating to GHB/GBL withdrawal, it is suggested that the principles of the psycho-social model should be applied in post-detoxification planning.

Current research does not support the effectiveness of one psycho-social intervention over others in the case of GHB/GBL detoxification.

13.7 Health Harms from Repeated Use

13.7.1 Cognitive Effects

Regular GHB users can experience multiple comas as a result of frequent accidental overdosing. A study has found that repeated GHB-induced comas, but not GHB use per se, are associated with a possible negative effect on associative long-term memory processing and performance, although no causal link was established. The authors argue that this suggests that prevention and harm-reduction messages should address the damage associated with GHB-induced comas, even though GHB users who experience loss of consciousness do not experience other immediate adverse effects.[126]

13.7.2   GHB/GBL Dependence

GHB/GBL has a high dependence liability, with some users describing rapidly developing tolerance. Dependent users will often consume multiple daily doses, up to hourly in cases of severe dependence, and this pattern can establish itself within as little as a few weeks of regular use. Dependent users can experience the rapid onset of withdrawal symptoms,[111] often between 30 minutes and a few hours after last dose (but these can also occur up to 48 hours after last use).

13.8   Management of Health Harms from Repeated Use

The management of GHB/GBL dependence is complex and the most appropriate approach will depend on the patient's identified goals – broadly, abstinence versus attempted controlled use. It is suggested that the management of GHB/GBL dependence should follow the established approach used for other drugs and include consideration of biological, psychological and social interventions. At present there are no specific interventions for GHB/GBL dependence supported by the research literature.

Interventions should consider the context of GHB use, particularly as GHB/GBL are sometimes used in a sexual context. Addressing the dependence is likely to require consideration of the impact of drug-facilitated sexual behaviours, sexual risk-taking and broader sexual health. This approach is often described as psychosexual therapy and can be an essential component of the overall treatment. Support in the safer use of geo-locating mobile telephone applications, which may be facilitators to meet sexual partners and buy drugs, should be considered.

As yet there is no evidence base upon which to recommend treatment for cognitive impairment related to GHB/GBL use, other than reducing or stopping use.

Depressant Drugs: Fentanyl, Fentanyl Analogues and Other Opioid NPS

14.1 Introduction

This chapter looks at the misuse of two groups of synthetic opioids. The first group includes fentanyl and fentanyl analogues; the second includes other novel synthetic opioids (opioid NPS). This chapter does not address issues pertaining to the use of these substances in legitimate therapeutic and clinical contexts.

In recent years, the use and harm caused by synthetic opioids has caused great concern, particularly in North America.

In addition to existing synthetic opioids, new opioids have emerged with structures distinct from those used therapeutically.

At a global level, it has been shown that the number of new synthetic opioid NPS (mostly fentanyl analogues) reported on drug markets has been rising at an unprecedented rate, from just 1 substance in 2009 to 46 by 2017. Synthetic opioids have become the second most important substance group, after stimulants, in terms of NPS reported for the first time. The group accounted for 29 per cent of the newly identified NPS in 2017. New synthetic opioid receptor agonists are dominated by newly emerging fentanyl analogues, and their number has risen markedly in recent years. Out of 78 NPS identified at the global level for the first time in 2017, forensic laboratories reported 22 new synthetic opioids receptor agonists, of which 19 were fentanyl analogues.[2]

In Europe, 49 new opioid NPS have been detected on the drug market since 2009, including 11 reported for the first time in 2018. The overall figure includes 34 fentanyl derivatives, 6 of which were reported for the first time in 2018. Although currently there appears to be a low prevalence of use, their increased availability and the fact that many are highly potent poses a serious threat to individual and public health.[6]

Included in this group are substances that have been 'rediscovered' by illicit manufacturers from previously published scientific literature. These substances were not developed as pharmaceutical agents at the time of their synthesis due to concerns about their potential toxicity. The group also contains newly designed opioid analogues produced by modifying the chemical structure of existing opioids in an attempt to avoid legal control.

14.2 Fentanyl and Fentanyl Analogues

14.2.1 Brief Pharmacology

Fentanyl (N-[1-(2-phenylethyl)-4-piperidinyl]-N-phenylpropanamide) is a potent and full agonist at the μ-opioid receptor. It has analgesic and sedative effects and is widely used in the management of severe pain and in anaesthesia. It is at least 80 times more potent than morphine, and when misused is associated with a high risk of acute toxicity. A number of non-pharmaceutical fentanyls have been detected in recent years.[127] [128] [129]

In comparison to heroin, fentanyls have a faster onset of action but a shorter duration of effect. When injected, fentanyls have an almost immediate effect, but maximal analgesic and respiratory depressant effect may not be noted for several minutes. The duration of action of fentanyl, when administered intravenously, is 30–60 minutes, much shorter than for heroin (4–5 hours). This may lead to frequent re-dosing.[130] Following intramuscular administration, the onset of action is from 7 to 8 minutes and the duration of action is 1–2 hours.

14.2.2 Mode of Use

Medical synthetic opiates, such as fentanyl, are available as patches, tablets, lollipops and solutions for injection. Fentanyls and other synthetic opioids like AH-7921 and MT-45 have been sold on drug markets as white powder.

Illicitly sourced fentanyl, mixed with heroin or other drugs, is driving unprecedented numbers of overdose deaths in some countries. There are reports from the USA and elsewhere of fentanyls being sold as, or mixed with, other illicit drugs,[131] including cocaine, crack cocaine, MDMA[162] and synthetic cannabinoid receptor agonists. Reports also suggest the adulteration of counterfeit prescription medication such as oxycodone and alprazolam with fentanyl and its analogues.[132] These reports suggest that many users are unaware that they are consuming fentanyls.

In the UK, fentanyl and fentanyl analogues are typically mis-sold on the illicit market as heroin, either substituted for heroin or mixed with it. There is little evidence of the direct marketing of fentanyl to drug users. As a result, when fentanyl is consumed, the end user usually believes that they have ingested heroin. Despite this, at the time of writing, fentanyl is infrequently detected in UK and European drug markets, in marked contrast to North America.

In some countries, however, fentanyl is sometimes diverted from pharmaceutical products, mostly extracted from transdermal patches, and to a lesser extent lozenges, sublingual tablets and solutions of fentanyl intended for infusion.

14.2.3 Desired Effects by User

Desired effects are similar to other opioids and include analgesia, anxiolysis, euphoria, drowsiness and feelings of relaxation.[133]

14.2.4   Acute Health Harms

Although there is a large body of evidence on the potential harms of pharmaceutical fentanyl, the evidence for the many fentanyl analogues is currently limited.

Nevertheless, although the acute toxicity of fentanyl analogues in humans has not been fully described, available evidence suggest that they are likely to be similar to established opioids, with considerable risk of acute toxicity, particularly respiratory depression.[134]

Acute Adverse Health Effects: Fentanyl and Analogues

- Features of fentanyl toxicity include: miosis (constriction of pupils or 'pinned' pupils), nausea and vomiting, anxiety, agitation, euphoria, depressed mood, persecutory thinking and hallucinations.

- Features of severe fentanyl toxicity include decreased consciousness, apnoea, and respiratory and central nervous system depression. Fentanyl overdose can lead to deep coma, convulsions and respiratory arrest. Sudden onset chest wall rigidity, sometimes referred to as 'wooden chest', may be associated with increased risk of mortality.

- The high potency of fentanyls, as well as their rapid onset of action, contributes to making them dangerous in a non-clinical context, particularly in comparison with heroin.[135]

Fentanyl overdose can begin suddenly, rapidly progress to death and manifest atypical physical symptoms. In comparison with heroin overdose, where death typically does not occur until at least 20–30 minutes after use, fentanyl in a non-clinical context can be associated with potentially lethal respiratory depression within 2 minutes.[136]

14.3   Other Opioid NPS (Excluding Fentanyls)

In recent years, a number of other synthetic opioids with structures distinct from those used in medical practice have entered the illicit market. These are typically produced in clandestine laboratories. Examples include, but are not limited to, the opioid analgesics, AH-7921 (a benzamide), U-47700 (a compound closely related to AH-7921) and MT-45 (a piperazine derivative)

14.3.1   Brief Pharmacology

AH-7921 acts act mainly as a μ-opioid receptor agonist,[137] as does U-47700, which is structurally related to AH-7921.[138] The latter also exhibits some k-opioid receptor agonism. The pharmacology of MT-45 is complex and involves opioid and non-opioid receptors that have not been fully characterised.[139]

14.3.2 Modes of Use

Opioid NPS are generally found on websites selling so-called 'research chemicals'.

They are consumed orally and sold as powder, tablets or capsules, [140] [141] but may also be consumed by inhalation/vaporising, nasal insufflation, sublingually, intravenous injection or rectal administration

User reports of opioid NPS suggest that the duration of effects of AH-7921 is approximately 4 hours, with a peak after 1.5 hours.[142] [143] The short duration of action of U-47700 was described by users to be associated with a very high urge to re-dose.[144] It appears that MT-45 has a slower onset of action, greater than 1–2 hours when taken orally, which may increase the risk of overdose from re-dosing before the peak effect is reached.[145]

14.3.3 Desired Effects by User

According to user reports, the effects of opioid NPS resemble those of classical opioids, including mild euphoria and relaxation. However, there are differences in effects from commonly used opioids, and from heroin in particular. AH-7921 and MT-45 have been reported to have intense dissociative effects, increase energy, reduce inhibition and increase sociability.[146] [139]

14.3.4 Acute Health Harms

The effects of non-fentanyl opioid NPS are broadly effects typical of opioid toxicity. Most are associated with miosis, with the exception of MT-45, which has only a small miotic effect. The small miotic effect of MT-45 in contrast to other commonly used opioid drug needs to be considered when undertaking clinical assessment[147] as clinicians may wrongly dismiss opioid use. Another unique feature of MT-45 toxicity is its association with ototoxicity leading to hearing loss.[148]

Overall, however, the effects of opioid NPS are broadly effects typical of opioid toxicity. They include itching and skin irritation, abdominal pain, constipation, urinary retention, light-headedness, headache, visual impairment, vertigo induced by movement, temperature change, tremors, numbness, seizures, hypertension and tachycardia.[140] [149] It is believed that non-fentanyl opioid NPS have a broadly similar or higher potential than morphine to cause severe acute adverse health effects. These effects include respiratory depression, hypothermia and withdrawal (in dependent users).[142] [150]

14.4 Case 8 Fentanyl Overdose

Presenting Complaint/History
A passer-by reports a man slumped against a wall in a side street.

Assessment
An ambulance is called and on arriving at the scene the crew find a man in his 40s, collapsed and unresponsive. There is a syringe nearby. On examination, the man has multiple old and fresh injection sites on both arms. GCS is 3 with BP of 80/45 and pulse of 42/min. Pupils are pinpoint. Respiratory rate is 8 breaths per minute and his SpO2 is 90% on room air.

Management
An opioid overdose is diagnosed and naloxone is administered. The man is transferred by ambulance to the nearest Emergency Department. His clinical presentation remains unchanged and a second dose of naloxone is administered.

This leads to some improvement, with the man regaining consciousness, his pulse and blood pressure stabilising and his ventilation improving. He is soon able to confirm his date of birth and a search of the hospital records reveals that he has regularly attended the Emergency Department over the last two years with multiple heroin overdoses. Over the next few minutes, however, he becomes drowsy and loses consciousness again. A naloxone infusion is commenced. His ventilation improves and observations normalise. He recovers sufficiently to sit up and talk. He explains that he was given heroin by his dealer but told to be careful as it was strong and showed the staff a small plastic packet of whitish powder, which he said he no longer wanted to use. The sample was sent for analysis and a few days later the results showed that it contained a number of different substances, notably fentanyl mixed with diamorphine.

Key Learning
There is evidence that potent opioid NPS, including fentanyl and its analogues, have been used as adulterants to 'street' heroin.

Fentanyl overdose should follow the same treatment protocols as used for heroin overdose. Additional doses of naloxone or a naloxone infusion may be needed due to the unpredictable potency and length of action of some opioid NPS. Note naloxone is given primarily to restore normal ventilation as opioids are such potent respiratory depressants.

14.5 Management of Acute Health Harms of Fentanyls and Other Opioid NPS

Naloxone

There is strong evidence that the prompt administration of the opioid receptor antagonist naloxone can reverse fentanyl-induced respiratory depression.

Extensive guidance has been issued in the UK on the provision of naloxone for the reversal of opioid overdoses in the community. Public Health England recommends that standard naloxone dosing (400 mcg doses repeated until breathing is restored) should sufficiently reverse the effects of an opioid overdose – even of a potent opioid – until an ambulance arrives.[151]

If there is suspicion that fentanyl is implicated in an overdose, it is essential that an ambulance or emergency services are called and transfer to hospital is promptly arranged. This is particularly important if naloxone is not available, or if the patient has not responded to repeated naloxone administration.

Basic resuscitation approaches (such as chest compressions and automatic defibrillators) may be required, particularly if responsiveness to naloxone administration is inadequate or delayed.[152]

14.6 Health Harms from Repeated Use of Fentanyls and Other Opioid NPS

Dependence

Fentanyls are associated with dependence, including tolerance and withdrawal symptoms similar to those reported with other opioids. Characteristic withdrawal symptoms include sweating, anxiety, diarrhoea, bone pain, abdominal cramps, shivers and 'goose flesh'.[153]

Despite limited information on the long-term use of other non-fentanyl opioid NPS, it can be assumed that they have a high dependence potential similar to morphine. Reports from users suggest tolerance can develop rapidly, and in dependent individuals withdrawal-like symptoms are similar to other opioids.

14.7 Management of Health Harms from Repeated Use of Fentanyls and Other Opioid NPS

In the absence of evidence to suggest otherwise, the treatment of dependence on fentanyl and other non-fentanyl opioid NPS should follow protocols for established opioids. In particular, treatment should be based on the principles and framework of the UK guidelines on the clinical management of drug misuse and dependence,[154] and should adhere to the recommendations of the reviews, technical appraisals, standards and national guidelines produced by the National Institute for Health and Care Excellence (NICE).[155]

Chapter 15

Depressant Drugs: Benzodiazepine NPS

15.1 Introduction and Brief Pharmacology

Benzodiazepines act as positive allosteric modulators on the GABA-A receptor, increasing the action of the inhibitory neurotransmitter GABA. Consumption of benzodiazepines can lead to psychoactive effects such as sedation and relaxation.

A concerning recent emerging pattern has been the increased availability and consumption of non-prescribed pharmaceutical and non-pharmaceutical benzodiazepines (benzodiazepine NPS).

Many of these uncontrolled benzodiazepine-type substances were NPS. However, in comparison to other types of NPS that have appeared in the last decade, the number of benzodiazepine NPS is small. The World Drug Report 2019 noted that out of the 492 drugs classified as NPS that were reported in 2017, only 25 were NPS with a sedative-hypnotic effect. Among all NPS reported in 2017, 79 were reported for the first time this year, and this only included 4 drugs with a sedative-hypnotic effect. Most such NPS are benzodiazepines, some of which have been patented, but many have never been marketed for medical use. The majority have never undergone clinical trials and are typically sold as 'legal benzodiazepines', 'designer benzodiazepines' or 'research chemicals'.[2]

Similarly in Europe, the overall number of benzodiazepine NPS is low, with the European Drug Report 2019 noting that the EMCDDA is monitoring 28 new benzodiazepines – 23 of which were first detected in Europe in the last 5 years. However, although the numbers are small, it is significant that over the last few years there has been an increase in the number, type and availability of new psychoactive substances belonging to the benzodiazepine class which are not controlled by international drug control laws. The World Drug Report suggests that this increase, as well as the similar increase in the number of opioid NPS, potentially signals that new psychoactive substances are increasingly more targeted at the long-term and more problematic drug users.[2]

In Europe, benzodiazepine NPS are sold as fake versions of commonly prescribed anti-anxiety medicines such as alprazolam (Xanax) and diazepam, making use of existing distribution networks in the illicit drug market. They are sold online, sometimes under their own names, and marketed as 'legal' versions of authorised medicines.[2]

There are broadly three different types of benzodiazepines being sold on the illicit market, and it is often difficult for the user to distinguish them.

- Pharmaceutically manufactured benzodiazepines, which are diverted from legitimate sources (e.g. diazepam in the UK, phenazepam and etizolam licensed in other countries).

- Counterfeit or adulterated benzodiazepines with unpredictable chemical content and strength. There are reports of 'super-strong' counterfeit 'Xanax', with much greater potency than the genuine pharmaceutical product, or illicit products containing different drugs, including other types of benzodiazepines or opioids.[156 157]

- Benzodiazepine NPS including drugs that have not been licensed as medications (in any country) but which are instead specifically manufactured for the illicit drug market. Generally sold on the internet as 'research chemicals', they have often been previously synthesised as potential drug candidates by pharmaceutical companies, but were not subsequently marketed as medication. Examples include diclazepam, flubromazepam, pyrazolam, clonazolam, deschloroetizolam, flubromazolam, nifoxipam and meclonazepam. It can be assumed that many more will appear.

15.2 Modes of Use

Benzodiazepine NPS are available as tablets, capsules, powders and on blotters (similar to LSD).[158] Irrespective of form, the content can vary greatly in terms of active ingredient(s), making it difficult for users to measure doses accurately and leading to the risk of unintended overdose.

15.3 Desired Effects by User

Benzodiazepine NPS are used recreationally on their own or combined with other drugs and/or alcohol. The desired effects include relaxation and somnolence or to moderate the unwanted effects of other drugs, such as stimulant-induced insomnia. Benzodiazepine NPS may also be used to manage the symptoms of mental health problems such as anxiety, insomnia and low mood.

15.4 Acute Health Harms

Knowledge of non-pharmaceutical benzodiazepine NPS is limited; however, it is probable that their acute adverse health effects will be similar to those currently seen in pharmaceutical benzodiazepines and will require similar clinical management.

Acute adverse health effects include impaired coordination, confusion, excessive drowsiness, coma and respiratory arrest. Withdrawal symptoms including agitation and drug craving are seen in dependent users upon reduction or cessation of use.

The limited evidence available on the benzodiazepine NPS suggests that some of the newer substances have either a higher potency and/or longer duration of action than traditional benzodiazepines, which in turn may lead to increased risks to the user. For example, there is emerging evidence of severe intoxication following the use of flubromazolam, resulting in prolonged, severe symptoms including hypotension, rhabdomyolysis and coma.[159]

Similarly, etizolam has an estimated potency five times greater than diazepam and is sometimes sold dried onto blotting paper, making it very difficult for the user to estimate the dose.

15.5 Management of Acute Health Harms

In the absence of evidence to suggest otherwise, the treatment of benzodiazepine NPS harms should follow protocols used for established benzodiazepines. In the case of severe intoxication, the GABA antagonist flumazenil should be considered in accordance with local/national protocols.

15.6 Health Harms from Repeated Use

Many benzodiazepine NPS have a significant dependence liability, which may be greater than that of existing pharmaceutical benzodiazepines. Other harms related to longer-term use of benzodiazepine NPS are currently poorly understood.

15.7 Management of Health Harms from Repeated Use

As with all drug misuse problems, no single approach is likely to be sufficient. A consideration of biological, psychological and social factors is suggested, including careful attention to genetic vulnerabilities, current mental and physical health and the social context of drug use.

Depressant Drugs: Ketamine and Its Analogues

16.1 Introduction

Ketamine is not a new psychoactive substance; it has been produced as a pharmaceutical product for many decades. It is a licensed anaesthetic and analgesic medication in many countries and is particularly used in paediatric, emergency and veterinary medicine. Ketamine appears to possess rapid antidepressant effects, independent of its transient psychoactive effects. There is increasing evidence that ketamine may have therapeutic uses for the management of treatment-resistant depression and post-traumatic stress disorder.[160 161]

This section will look at the illicit use of ketamine and its analogues and the associated risks, particularly in the light of evidence of increased prevalence of recreational use. It will not address issues in relation to the medicinal use of ketamine by professionals in clinical settings.

Ketamine and its analogues are sometimes described as 'dissociative' drugs. The term 'dissociative' is used to describe a state of sensory loss and analgesia, as well as amnesia, which is not accompanied by actual loss of consciousness. Ketamine has the capacity to induce an emotional state in which users often describe their consciousness as being separated from their body. It can lead to a trance-like cataleptic state, amnesia and deep analgesia, but with intact ocular, laryngeal and pharyngeal reflexes.

16.2 Brief Pharmacology

16.2.1 Ketamine

Ketamine and its analogues are predominantly sedative drugs, with a complex neuro-chemical profile, reflecting their actions as psychostimulant, dissociative, anaesthetic and analgesic substances, with amnestic properties.

Ketamine is a non-competitive NMDA receptor antagonist and also shows affinity for mu, delta, and sigma opioid receptors and monoamine transporters. Ketamine also acts at dopamine D2 and $5\text{-}HT_{2A}$ receptors, and the activation of 5-HT$_{2A}$ receptors is thought to be related to ketamine's resulting perceptual and hallucinogenic effects.

16.2.2 Methoxetamine

Methoxetamine is a ketamine analogue. It is both a dopamine reuptake inhibitor and an NMDA receptor blocker. Its affinity for the NMDA receptor is comparable to or higher than that of ketamine. Methoxetamine also has affinity for the serotonin transporters.[162]

16.3 Modes of Use

Ketamine is available on the illicit drug market in two main forms. The first is pharmaceutical ketamine diverted from medicinal supplies. In the UK this is relatively rare. Much more common is illicitly manufactured ketamine with variable purity and numerous adulterants.

Illicitly manufactured ketamine is typically sold in the form of a powder or fine crystal, but may also be available as tablets. Ketamine powder is typically insufflated (snorted), but it can be injected.

Methoxetamine is generally sold as a white crystal powder, but can be found in tablet form. It is generally used by insufflation, but can be used orally (as tablets or the powder wrapped in a cigarette paper and swallowed), sublingually, rectally and by injection.

16.4 Desired Effects by User

Ketamine can produce a range of dose-dependent effects, although effects may also be influenced by other factors, including the individual's tolerance, other drugs ingested and setting of use.[163]

In general:

- At low doses, ketamine can cause relaxation, distortion of time and space, visual and auditory hallucinations and mild dissociative effects. It can also have stimulant-type properties.[164]
- At high doses, ketamine produces more pronounced dissociation, where the user experiences feelings of intense detachment. Perceptions can appear completely separated from reality. This is sometimes referred to by users as the 'k-hole'.

The effects of ketamine are generally short-lived, typically lasting up to 1 hour. This short duration of effect may promote repeated dosing to maintain effects over time.

The intended effects of methoxetamine are similar to those of ketamine; however, the effects last longer and the onset is delayed in comparison to ketamine.[165]

16.5 Acute Health Harms

Ketamine can cause unconsciousness, amnesia and analgesia, while maintaining relative haemodynamic stability, even when large doses are consumed. Clinical features of acute intoxication are typically dose dependent.

Features of acute ketamine intoxication can include:[166]

- Dissociative-type symptoms, distortions and hallucinations (visual and auditory)
- Persecutory thinking and psychotic states (typically short-lived with complete resolution). In patients with schizophrenia stabilised on an antipsychotic, ketamine can cause a relapse of psychosis.
- Significant analgesia, slurred speech, dizziness, numbness, confusion, blurred vision, insomnia, decreased sexual motivation, impairments in working and episodic memory.[167]
- Ataxia, agitation, aggression.
- Cardiovascular effects, including sinus tachycardia, hypertension, chest pain, palpitations and pulmonary oedema. Cardiovascular effects can be severe, especially for people with hypertension, severe cardiac disease or at risk of stroke. Risks are increased with co-ingestion of stimulants.[168] Ketamine is a derivative of phencyclidine (PCP), and, like PCP, ketamine stimulates cardiac and respiratory function, although it is less toxic and shorter acting than PCP.
- There are some reports of raised intracranial pressure, polyneuropathy and seizures, but these appear relatively rare.

Although rare, it is possible that respiratory depression can happen in the context of overdose. However, even when a user is very intoxicated, the coughing and swallowing reflexes are maintained, with minor suppression of the gag reflex.

The features of acute intoxication can make ketamine users vulnerable to accidents. The adverse effects of ketamine can be related to its dissociative properties and other features of acute intoxication. These can have a profound effect on the user's ability to function. Analgesia can lead users to be unaware that they have suffered serious or even life-threatening injury. Other risks include falls, drowning or assault by others while intoxicated.

16.6 Management of Acute Health Harms

The effects of ketamine toxicity develop rapidly and are generally short-lived, with most patients improving rapidly.[169][170]

No antidote exists for ketamine overdose. The management of acute ketamine toxicity is supportive care.

Observation of the patient until vital signs and mental state have normalised is recommended. It is suggested that in order to prevent excessive agitation a person with acute intoxication is removed from unnecessary auditory and visual stimulation until the symptoms resolve. Benzodiazepines may be required.

Management should also include appropriate assessment of co-ingestion of other psychoactive drugs, head injury or hypoglycaemia. It is suggested that if symptoms fail to improve within an hour of presentation, the diagnosis and management should be reviewed.[171]

Profoundly obtunded patients may require airway support, intravenous fluids and titrated benzodiazepine therapy if they are agitated, hyperthermic or show overt sympathomimetic signs.[172]

16.7 Health Harms from Repeated Use

16.7.1 Effects on Cognitive Function

Frequent and long-term ketamine use can be associated with neurocognitive impairment, in particular working and episodic memory, semantic processing and visual recognition.[173] [174]

16.7.2 Dependence and Withdrawal

Frequent ketamine use is associated with tolerance.[175]

There are reports of ketamine dependence[176] and psychological withdrawal symptoms.[177] These include anxiety, shaking, sweating, palpitations, 'chills', autonomic arousal, lacrimation, restlessness, nightmares, drug hunting, tiredness, low appetite and low mood.[178]

16.7.3 Physical Long-Term and Chronic Harms

The use of ketamine has been associated with damage to the urinary tract, although the aetiology is poorly understood.

Ketamine use is associated with damage that can affect the entire urinary tract, and with ulcerative cystitis[168] in particular being recognised. Damage can be severe, and in some cases irreversible.[179]

The urological syndrome associated with ketamine use includes dysuria, haematuria, polyuria, urge incontinence, nocturia, obstruction of the upper urinary tract, papillary necrosis and renal dysfunction. Ulceration of the bladder wall can lead to scarring, which in turn reduces bladder function and can, when severe, require reconstructive surgery.[180] The severe pain resulting from ketamine-induced urinary tract damage can be a barrier to abstinence from ketamine. Users will self-medicate with further ketamine, aware that the drug's analgesic effects temporarily control their distress. Continued use of ketamine aggravates both the bladder damage and substance use disorder. Although the ketamine analogue methoxetamine is sometimes promoted on the illicit market as a 'bladder friendly' alternative to ketamine, there is some evidence that methoxetamine can induce changes in the kidney and bladder after daily use, suggesting that chronic use of methoxetamine in humans may be associated with similar lower urinary tract symptoms as those described for chronic ketamine use.[181]

People with long-term and heavy use of ketamine have reported intense abdominal pain (referred to by some users in the UK as 'k-cramps'). Symptoms appear to resolve once the patient stops using ketamine. The cause is not well understood.[182]

16.8 Case 9 Ketamine Bladder

Presenting Complaint/History

Rachel is a 26-year-old accounts manager living with two flatmates in Exeter. Her job is highly stressful and Rachel frequently returns home 'exhausted' and 'stressed'. Her boss is often critical of her work and in the last few months Rachel has become increasingly anxious, often waking with a feeling of dread. When she was 21 and sitting her finals at university, Rachel experienced a similar feeling and was eventually prescribed antidepressants for a few months by her GP, which she felt helped her.

While at university, Rachel used MDMA and occasionally cocaine, and drank around 40 SAU a week during this period. She felt that these amounts were no more or less than her friends consumed.

Since starting work, Rachel has reduced her alcohol consumption considerably and now typically drinks 6 SAU, once a week. She has also reduced her illicit drug consumption and no longer uses cocaine or MDMA. Instead, Rachel uses ketamine, which she first tried about one year ago. The effects of ketamine seem to Rachel to be quite different from the other drugs she had tried. Ketamine makes Rachel feel 'relaxed', 'numb' and unconcerned with her worries. Rachel initially used ketamine while clubbing with friends but now uses it at home on her own. If she has experienced a particularly difficult day at work, she will tell herself that she deserves a 'treat' and consume ketamine. As the job has become more stressful, her usage has increased. Rachel now uses 'a little bit' of ketamine 'most days' but is aware that she now needs to use more of the drug to experience the same benefits. She estimates that she is now consuming around 6gm per week, which she buys online and which arrives by post.

Over the last month, Rachel has begun to experience lower abdominal pain. She described discomfort when urinating, saying it sometimes 'burns'. She also described significant polyuria, often needing to urinate every 20–30 minutes. Rachel's work colleagues have noticed this, as she often needs to leave meetings three or four times. Rachel went to see her GP, who took a urine specimen and told her that there was a trace of blood and that she most likely had a urinary tract infection. Rachel did not tell the GP about her ketamine use as she felt embarrassed. Antibiotics were prescribed, which Rachel took for one week without benefit and decided not to return to see the GP. Over the next few weeks, however, her symptoms worsened considerably. The pain on micturition increased, to the point where it feels like 'peeing broken glass'. Rachel also notices that her urine is darker than usual and that she has a constant dull ache over her bladder. The only thing that improves the symptoms is taking ketamine, which provides up to half an hour of relief. Rachel starts to use small amounts of ketamine during her coffee and lunch breaks to keep the pain under control, but is aware that her performance at work is deteriorating as a result. She is now consuming around 12 grams per week.

Not knowing what to do, Rachel looks up her symptoms on the internet. She is worried that she might have bladder cancer. She finds several articles suggesting that ketamine can cause bladder damage and Rachel decides to stop using ketamine completely to see if that will help. The following day she goes to work and leaves the ketamine at home. By mid-morning she is feeling very uncomfortable; her urine, which had been dark for several weeks, now contains what look like blood clots. Her work colleagues notice Rachel's distress and ask if she is feeling alright. Rachel says she has flu and is now desperate to return home and take ketamine to make the pain go away. Once home, Rachel takes 2gm of ketamine (much more than she would usually use in one go) and soon feels the pain ease. She makes an emergency appointment with her GP and tells them about the ketamine use and her fear that it may be causing the bladder symptoms. The GP starts a second course of antibiotics and refers Rachel to both the local drug service and urology department.

Assessment

In the course of her drug misuse assessment, Rachel is asked to complete a screening tool for bladder symptoms. She is diagnosed with ketamine dependence as well as ketamine-related urological symptoms. Rachel identifies abstinence from ketamine as her treatment goal. Subsequent review by the urology team, including cystoscopy, confirms ulcerative cystitis resulting from ketamine use.

Management

The drug treatment and urology team work in partnership to establish a treatment plan for Rachel. The first step is to agree a pain management plan to treat the ulcerative cystitis. The drug treatment team are reluctant for opioids to be prescribed given their dependence-forming properties and so NSAIDs are used. Fortunately Rachel responds well to this medication and finds that she no longer need to use ketamine to control her pain.

Rachel engages in drug treatment and makes good progress in reducing her quantity and frequency of use. She engages particularly well with psychological work and says that she wants to address the anxiety which she feels has been present for many years. She commences cognitive behavioural therapy with a specific focus on anxiety management.

Two months later, Rachel has not used ketamine for five weeks. The urology team have reassured her that as long as she does not return to using ketamine, her bladder should fully recover. The drug treatment service focuses particularly on helping Rachel develop relapse prevention strategies.

Key Learning
Ketamine can cause significant and debilitating urological tract damage.

Symptoms can often be mistaken for urinary tract infections and incorrectly treated with antibiotics.

Paradoxically, users will often consume ketamine as an analgesic to bring temporary relief from the ketamine-induced bladder symptoms. A pain management plan, agreed between urology and drug treatment services, is indicated.

Most ketamine users who experience urological damage make a full recovery with cessation of use. However, there are cases in which surgical repair or even cystectomy has been required.

16.9   Management of Health Harms from Repeated Use

16.9.1   Urological Intervention
People who use ketamine and experience recurrent urological problems or unexplained urinary symptoms should be assessed by a specialist drug treatment service and, where relevant, referred to an urologist.

Abstinence from ketamine is essential. If drug cessation is achieved, the urological symptoms may be partially or completely reversed, but if ketamine use persists, so do the symptoms. Strategies are limited when ketamine use continues.[183]

In some people, symptoms will persist despite stopping ketamine use.

Treatment for urinary tract symptoms and ketamine-induced uropathy has been described as either symptomatic (analgesia, urinary diversion) or the treatment of complications (e.g. percutaneous nephrostomy insertion).

Frequent ketamine users may have irreversible damage and scarring. The most affected patients may require major surgery, in the form of cystectomy and bladder reconstruction.[180]

The need for pain control in patients with ulcerative cystitis should be considered as users may self-medicate with ketamine. Clinical experience suggests that substance misuse clinicians are advised to work jointly with urology services to ensure that a pain management plan is in place.

Chapter

17

Synthetic Cannabinoid Receptor Agonists (SCRAs)

17.1 Introduction

Synthetic Cannabinoid Receptor Agonists (SCRAs) are a diverse group of substances that act on the same brain receptors as tetrahydrocannabinol (THC), the main psychoactive ingredient of cannabis. Some SCRAs also work at other receptors. They are sold in a wide range of strengths and are sometimes referred to using the name of branded products such as 'Spice' or 'Mamba' in the UK and 'K2' in North America.

SCRAs were first developed for the illicit market to mimic the effects of natural cannabis and to appeal to natural cannabis users. However, despite this they have tended to be most commonly used by vulnerable groups, such as the homeless and prisoners, where their appeal appears to be that they are cheap and potent intoxicants.[2]

A large number of different types of SCRAs exist, with some having significantly stronger effects than others. Synthetic cannabinoids represent the largest group of substances currently monitored in Europe by the EMCDDA through the EU Early Warning System. Among all NPS reported to UNODC by the end of 2017, synthetic cannabinoids constitute the largest category of substances reported.[1] In Europe, 179 SCRAs were detected from 2008 to 2017, including 10 reported in 2017. The smoking of synthetic cannabinoids in marginalised populations, including among homeless people and prisoners, has been identified by the 2019 European Drug Report as a problem in a number of European countries.[6]

17.2 Brief Pharmacology

SCRAs are a large, chemically diverse group of molecules with some functional similarity to natural THC, as well as to other phytocannabinoids. However, there is little structural similarity between most SCRAs and THC or other naturally occurring cannabinoids.

Both SCRAs and natural cannabis (THC) bind to the CB1 receptors. SCRAs often have a much stronger agonism for CB1 receptors than natural cannabis, resulting in the greater psychoactive effect of many SCRAs. Some SCRAs are much more potent and potentially more toxic than THC.

In contrast to natural cannabis, SCRAs do not contain cannabidiol (CBD), thought to possess anxiolytic, anti-psychotic and anti-craving properties. It has been suggested that the presence of CBD reduces the risk of THC-induced psychosis in natural cannabis.[184] As SCRAs do not contain CBD, their risk of causing psychosis is argued to be greater.

There are important differences between the various SCRAs. Products containing SCRAs can range from those with potency similar to THC to those that are significantly stronger.[185]

The major SCRA groups include the HU series (developed at the Hebrew University), the CP series (from Pfizer Inc.) and the JWH series (developed by JW Huffman).

New generations of SCRAs have developed over the years, including those based on modifications of a 'model' compound (JWH-018, for example). More recent formulations (referred to as 'third-' or 'fourth generation') are typically more potent than earlier generations of SCRAs and may be associated with greater clinical harms.

SCRAs, including AMB-FUBINACA, ADB-CHMINACA, ABCHMINACA, MDMB-CHMICA and AB-FUBINACA, are associated with severe adverse reactions, serious toxicity and death.[186] Other SCRAS have also been linked to 'bizarre' behaviour, such as stereotypical movements and acute psychotic effects.[187]

17.3 Modes of Use

Most of the synthetic cannabinoid products used for recreational purposes in the UK are produced by taking an inert herbal product then spraying it with one or more SCRAs before drying and packaging it for the user to smoke. In this way, SCRAs are produced in a form familiar to natural cannabis users. Users are likely to find it difficult to distinguish one SCRA from another as many products will look similar even if they contain very different SCRAs.

SCRAs can also be sprayed onto tobacco or paper, or impregnated into textiles. There is anecdotal evidence that postal packages, letters or clothes sprayed with SCRAs have been used to bring drugs into prisons.

More recently, SCRA-containing products appear to be diversifying. At a European level, the EMCDDA has reported SCRAs in products that look like cannabis resin, either in branded 'legal high' products or mis-sold to unknowing customers as cannabis resin on the illicit market.

SCRAs have also been detected in mixtures containing other NPS, such as stimulants, hallucinogens and sedative/ hypnotics. In Hungary and the United

States, synthetic cannabinoids have been detected in what appear to be ecstasy tablets, leading to clusters of acute poisonings. Recently, there has been anecdotal information regarding the use of SCRAs in liquid form being consumed using e-cigarettes.[188]

17.4 Desired Effects by User

Although SCRAs produce effects similar to those produced by THC, they are not the same. Desired effects include relaxation, euphoria, perceptual distortions and hallucinations. However, along with generally greater potency, some SCRAs may have long half-lives, leading to much more prolonged and intense psychoactive effects than would be typically experienced with natural cannabis.

17.5 Acute Health Harms

There is a wide range of adverse health effects reported following the consumption of SCRAs, with unpredictable effects ranging from profound sedation to intense agitation and psychosis.[158] Many of the reported adverse effects are in marked contrast to natural cannabis effects.

A number of user surveys suggest higher need for emergency medical care by those using SCRAs in comparison to natural cannabis, although these episodes appeared to largely require only symptomatic or supportive care and were of short duration.[189] In addition, SCRA use has been associated with increased levels of violence [190] and psychosis in the absence of a personal or family history of psychosis.[185 191 192 193]

17.5.1 Features of SCRA Toxicity Include:

Neurological, Cognitive and Psychiatric Effects

- Severe anxiety, agitation, aggressiveness, mood disturbance, suicidal thoughts, thought disorganisation, perceptional changes, persecutory thinking, delusions, auditory and visual hallucinations.
- Numbness, tingling, light-headedness, dizziness, pallor, tinnitus, diaphoresis, tremor, impaired motor performance, somnolence, syncope, nystagmus, convulsions, reduced levels of consciousness, catatonia, coma.
- Short-term memory and cognitive deficits, confusion, amnesia.

Cardiovascular/Cerebral Effects

- Tachycardia, hypertension, hypotension, hypokalaemia, chest pain, palpitations, myocardial ischaemia, myocardial infarction, ischaemic strokes

Neuromuscular and Musculoskeletal Effects
• Hypertonia, myoclonus, myalgia, rhabdomyolysis

Renal Effects
• Acute kidney injury (aetiology unknown)

Other Effects
• Hyperglycaemia, hypoglycaemia, respiratory acidosis, cold extremities, dyspnoea, mydriasis, nausea, vomiting, loss of sight and speech

Serotonin Syndrome
• Some SCRAs have been linked to the serotonin syndrome.

17.6 Case 10 'Spice Attack' in Prison

Presenting Complaint/History
Prison staff are called to an emergency in one of the cells after the alarm has been raised about an inmate, who is said to be having a 'spice attack' following the consumption of a SCRA.

Assessment
On entering the cell, a man is found standing in the corner looking preoccupied and distressed. There are several deep cuts on his arm, which appear to have been self-inflicted. On hearing his name, the man responds with verbal abuse and begins throwing objects at staff. In an attempt to de-escalate the situation, staff withdraw from the cell but continue to observe from outside. The injured man paces his cell several times, apparently talking to himself, before suddenly falling to the floor.

Staff, including the medical team, re-enter the cell and an ambulance is called.

The man now appears very drowsy but responds to his name being called. He is helped from the cell and taken to hospital.

During his transfer he receives standard assessment and supportive management, including securing IV access, assessment of blood sugar and close observation of vital signs.

Management
In hospital, he remains very drowsy but is able to support his own airway. Blood pressure is unremarkable, but there is a sinus tachycardia of 112 beats/min. His wounds are dressed and he is moved to Resus. Thirty minutes after being admitted to the Emergency Room, the man becomes agitated again. He emerges from the cubical holding a chair and shouts unintelligibly at staff. When staff try to reassure the man, he throws the chair, hitting a member of

staff on the arm, before lashing out at another patient. Security are called and five members of staff are needed to restrain the man. IM lorazepam is administered. The man becomes calmer, apologises for getting angry and once more becomes drowsy. Staff administer another small amount of lorazepam and continue to closely monitor him, with security in attendance.

Over the next two hours, the clinical presentation fluctuates rapidly between over-sedation and agitation, but the symptoms gradually reduce in intensity. Three hours after admission to the Emergency Room, the man is fully orientated and denies any perceptual disturbance. He reports that he had consumed 'spice' in his cell. ECG and routine bloods are unremarkable and a urine drug screen is negative for all drugs (but is unable to test for SCRAs). After a period of further observation he is returned to prison.

Key Learning

The use of SCRAs has been associated with a greater risk of psychiatric morbidity and psychosis than with natural cannabis.

Intoxication with SCRAs can result in a range of acute symptoms, including agitation, sedation and psychosis. Symptoms often fluctuate in intensity and can alternate from intense agitation to marked sedation.

Psychosis linked to SCRAs has been associated with more agitation than would typically be expected from natural cannabis alone.

SCRA-associated psychosis is typically transient, but some individuals may experience psychosis that persists for weeks after the acute intoxication.

SCRAs may precipitate psychosis in both vulnerable individuals and otherwise healthy people with no history of psychosis.

17.7 Management of Acute Health Harms

Acute SCRA intoxication is generally short-lived and self-limiting.[194] However, some people will present with SCRA-related adverse effects, which can be long-lasting and severe.

The management of SCRA toxicity is symptomatic and supportive, as no antidotes exist. Supportive treatment is dependent on a patient's specific presentation.

- Hydration and monitoring may be enough for patients with mild to moderate intoxication.[195]
- Benzodiazepines may be of benefit for patients who present with symptoms of anxiety, panic and agitation. Prescribing for agitation should only be short term.

- Anti-psychotic medication may be indicated for some patients, especially those who present with severe agitation or aggression, when the patient has a history of psychotic disorders, and when the psychotic symptoms do not remit spontaneously or with supportive care.[196]

In symptomatic patients, pulse and blood pressure should be monitored. In a minority of cases, SCRA consumption can be associated with severe cardiovascular, cerebrovascular, neurological, psychiatric and renal effects. Rhabdomyolysis and cardiac or cerebral ischaemia should be considered.

17.8 Health Harms from Repeated Use

The evidence of the adverse effects of prolonged SCRA use is still emerging. There is some evidence of persistent psychosis among those reported to use SCRAs frequently, and cognitive impairment has been described with daily use.

Although the evidence is currently limited, SCRAs may have greater dependence liability than natural cannabis, and this may develop more quickly. There are reports of withdrawal symptoms following frequent SCRA use, which can be severe and prolonged.[197]

17.8.1 Withdrawal Symptoms from SCRAs

A number of symptoms have been described in SCRA-dependent users who reduce or cease use of the drug. These include:

- Headaches
- Anxiety
- Coughing
- Insomnia/sleep disturbance
- Impatience, difficulty concentrating
- Anger/irritability
- Restlessness
- Nausea
- Depression
- Craving
- Diaphoresis
- Tremor
- Hypertension
- Tachycardia

The chemical diversity of SCRAs has made it difficult to build an accurate picture of the typical length and severity of withdrawals in dependent users.

17.9 Case 11 SCRA Dependence in Homeless Population

Presenting Complaint/History

Alfie is a 31-year-old man who has been sleeping on the street most nights for the last year. He has a previous history of heroin and alcohol dependence, but at present is not using either substance. Alfie thinks he has also been diagnosed with mental health problems in the past, stating that he thinks he may have 'bipolar', 'depression', 'ADD' and 'reading problems'.

Alfie asks to see one of the outreach workers because he is worried about his use of 'Mamba', and the worker meets with Alfie the following afternoon.

Assessment

Alfie tells the outreach worker than he started using Mamba after he was given it by a friend as 'a treat'. He smoked the drug with tobacco and liked the relaxing effect, stating that the drug 'calms my head'. Unfortunately, Alfie found the Mamba 'very moreish' and now thinks he is using too much. He agrees to meet with the local drug service for an assessment.

At this assessment, Alfie estimates that he has been smoking around 'one gram' of Mamba daily for the last six months. He typically smokes small doses every few hours. If he goes without smoking Mamba for more than six hours he experiences withdrawal symptoms, including sweating, shaking, drug craving and intense agitation. Alfie explained that he found these withdrawals to be 'worse than heroin'. He identified his treatment goal as complete abstinence from Mamba. He denies using any other drugs.

Management

Alfie agreed to attend appointments at the clinic to help him develop a plan to incrementally reduce his Mamba use. Unfortunately, he found it difficult to attend appointments regularly because he needed to move to different parts of the city to find somewhere to sleep. The team link Alfie with a number of homeless services who offer Alfie temporary hostel accommodation, but Alfie said he preferred to stay on the street because he was worried about people 'stealing my stuff'. It was unclear if this represented persecutory thinking or a valid fear based on previous experiences of being in hostels.

When Alfie did attend the clinic, he engaged well with staff and made intermittent progress in reducing his Mamba consumption. Progress was typically followed by significant relapse, and the team discussed with Alfie the option of an inpatient detoxification. Alfie refused this option as he did not want to be 'banged up in a prison', and despite offers for him to visit the inpatient unit to see if he would reconsider, Alfie declined. At his last appointment, Alfie told staff that he had completely stopped using Mamba and would not be using it again. Unfortunately, he achieved this by returning to dependent drinking and reported drinking around 20 standard alcohol units daily. He disengaged with the clinic, and despite attempts to re-contact him by the clinic and outreach services, Alfie is lost to follow up.

> **Key Learning**
>
> In the UK, the use of SCRAs is concentrated in homeless and prison populations. These populations have multiple complex needs and any treatment plan will need to consider issues such as housing, physical and mental health needs and substance misuse management.
>
> SCRAs can cause significant dependence, with marked tolerance and withdrawals symptoms.
>
> Withdrawal symptoms can be severe and there are reports of seizures.
>
> Management should follow treatment protocols for other substances, with a focus on enhancing motivation towards the treatment goal and addressing both substance use and co-morbidities. There is currently no substitution prescribing or antidote available for SCRAs.

17.10 Management of Health Harms from Repeated Use

The large number of SCRAs with different potencies coupled with a poor understanding by clinicians (and users) of what has been consumed has led to significant uncertainty about the longer-term harms of SCRAs and the best way to manage these harms. At present, the best advice appears to be cessation of use and appropriate management of other co-existing mental and physical health problems. Where psychosis has developed, antipsychotics may help. For dependent users, standard bio-psycho-social management is suggested until further research is available to guide best practice.

17.10.1 SCRAs in Prison

There is evidence that in a number of European countries, SCRAs are the most common group of NPS used in prison.[198] A UK study in 10 prisons found the prevalence of SCRA use among prisoners preparing for release to be twice the level measured among prisoners at the time of admission (16% testing positive versus 8% positive, respectively). It was the only substance for which the percentage of positive drug tests was higher pre-release than upon arrival in prison.[199]

The use of synthetic cannabinoids in prisons has been linked to a number of factors:

- It has been suggested that inmates use SCRAs to 'deaden time' in prison.[200]
- SCRAs and other NPS are also used in prison for self-medication purposes or as compensation for perceived under-medication. Self-medication to cope with feelings of depression and anxiety were reported. In this context, the reported powerful psychoactive effects of SCRAs appears to be important to prisoners.

- Dependence on SCRAs prior to entering prison has been identified as another motivation to continue to use, with some prisoners describing how their patterns of use were habitual.[201]
- It has also been reported that SCRAs may sometimes be used by those withdrawing from a dependence on other substances, such as heroin, when entering prison.[198]

Chapter

18

Hallucinogens

18.1 Introduction

Hallucinogens are a diverse group of drugs that alter and distort perception, producing sensory distortions (most typically visual, but possible in all modalities), and also modify thought and mood. They have large differences in psychoactive effect and potential adverse health effects.

There is increasing interest in the therapeutic use of hallucinogens in a controlled setting,[202] including for treatment-resistant depression,[203] and as a treatment for alcohol dependence,[204] smoking cessation,[205] anxiety and depression in life-threatening illnesses[206] and in palliative care.[207] Research is at an early stage, and more evidence is needed before recommendations can be made.

18.2 Brief Pharmacology

The term 'hallucinogen' is used in this section to refer to drugs with a mechanism of action mediated primarily by agonism of the 5-HT_{2A} receptors. The potency of hallucinogenic substances appears to be broadly, but not entirely, a function of affinity to the 5-HT_{2A} receptor. LSD, for example, has a high affinity with the 5-HT_{2A} receptor and is a potent hallucinogenic substance. Hallucinogenic drugs interact with other receptor sites too, contributing to the psychopharmacological and behavioural effects.

Tryptamines, phenethylamines and lysergamides form the three main groups of hallucinogenic drugs. A number of hallucinogen NPS have been reported in each of these groups, including:

- Ring-substituted phenethylamines (e.g. 2 C Series, and their derivatives. 2 C-B has various close analogues: bk-2 C-B, and 25B-NBOMe. The same selection of analogues may exist for the rest of the 2 C series, e.g. 2 C-E, 2 C-I, 2 C-T-7)

- Tryptamines (e.g. DMT, αMT, 5-MeO-DALT, DiPT, 5-MeO-DiPT)
- Lysergamides (e.g. ALD-52, ETH-LAD)

As with other psychoactive drugs, the effects of hallucinogens can vary greatly between different drugs and with different doses. For example, 2 C-B at lower doses causes heightened energy and empathy similar to that produced by MDMA, but at higher doses its effects are more similar to LSD.

Some drugs possess stimulant as well as hallucinogenic properties – for example, the NBOMes.[208] A recent small study on DMT reported significant increases in phenomenological features associated with near-death experience following DMT administration compared to placebos.[209]

As with other NPS, there have been consecutive generations of hallucinogen NPS. For example, 2C-B appeared on the drug market in the mid-1980s as a legal MDMA replacement. Its derivative, 25B-NBOMe, is a highly potent 2C-B derivative even at microgram-level doses.[210] NBOMes are also agonists for the alpha-adrenergic receptors. A number of hallucinogen NPS are highly potent at doses of milligrams or even micrograms.

Some hallucinogen NPS, such as the NBOMe series and bromo-dragonfly, are particularly potent and long-lasting. Researchers have speculated that users have found NBOMe too potent, resulting in limited use.[7]

18.3 Modes of Use

Hallucinogens are typically ingested orally, or sublingually, with the drug being dried onto small pieces of blotter paper or 'tabs', which are held in the mouth to allow absorption through the oral mucosa. Other less common routes of administration include insufflation, smoking, rectal and intravenous.

18.3.1 Onset and Length of Effects

Onset

The speed of onset of the effects of hallucinogen NPS differ widely and range from a few seconds to a few hours, depending on psychopharmacology and route of administration. For example, the effects of DMT will appear almost immediately, while those of LSD will begin approximately one hour after use. The effects of bromo-dragonfly may not be reached for up to 6 hours after ingestion, posing a risk that users re-dose under the mistaken belief that the first dose has had no effect. This is especially a risk where users wrongly believe they have taken a faster-acting hallucinogen.[211]

Duration of Effects

The duration of the effect of hallucinogens will also differ widely, ranging from:

- Very short effects (e.g. the effects of DMT will only last a few minutes)
- Intermediate duration of effects (e.g. 2C-B, with effects lasting 2–3 hours)
- Long duration (e.g. LSD and mescaline are longer-acting hallucinogens and a duration of 8–12 hours is common).
- Very long duration of effects (some NPS – including DOM and others in the DOx series, ibogaine, 2 C-P and bromo-dragonfly – have effects which have been reported to last a day or longer).[212]

There are often significant inter-individual differences in the effects of hallucinogen NPS depending on mental state at the time of consumption and the environment in which the drug is consumed. Non-pharmacological variables such as expectations, personality, environment and emotional state appear to have a greater influence on the effects of hallucinogens than with other drugs. In comparison with the more predictable and replicable effects of stimulants and depressants, the desired and actual effects of hallucinogen NPS are highly context-dependent and user-specific.

18.4 Desired Effects by User

Desired effects include euphoria, mild stimulation, enhanced appreciation of music and lights, visual distortions, intensification of sensual or sexual feelings and altered sense of time and place.

18.4.1 Microdosing

'Microdosing' is a term used for a pattern of consuming hallucinogens that has been growing in popularity and visibility. It refers to the use of a dose of hallucinogenic drug that is too small to cause intoxication or significant alteration of consciousness. The intention is that microdosing affects mood, health and cognition in positive ways, while allowing the user to carry on with everyday activities.[213]

It has been argued that taking small amounts of psilocybin mushrooms, LSD or mescaline enhances cognitive function, perception and creativity and adds a new dimension to what could be considered 'illegal cognitive enhancement'. This reflects a new desired effect of hallucinogenic drugs.[214] There is currently little evidence to draw upon regarding microdosing, although studies are proposed.[215]

The microdosing phenomenon has been spread most recently by the internet, where discussion fora enable users to share experiences and exchange information in ways that make new practices accessible to others. Its growing visibility has been reflected in substantial recent media coverage.

18.5 Acute Health Harms

18.5.1 Acute Intoxication

Effects on Mental Health

The most common cause of hospital presentations associated with the use of hallucinogen NPS is referred to by users as a 'bad trip'. This is best described as:

- Adverse psychological reaction occurring at typical doses.
- Common features include disturbing perceptions, intense dysphoria, anxiety, agitation and persecutory thinking.
- A patient's mental state may switch rapidly between severe anxiety and relative normality and back again.

At typical recreational doses, it is usual for people to maintain insight into the cause of their experiences, although the dread of 'permanent madness' or of death has been reported.[216] Hallucinogen NPS may provoke distressing thoughts and reflection on personal problems, past experiences and traumas.[217] They can profoundly exaggerate negative moods and depressed emotional states.[218]

Even when a user is not experiencing a 'bad trip', unwanted effects can include confusion, disorientation, anxiety and unwanted thoughts, emotions and memories. Hallucinogen NPS are only occasionally a cause of drug-induced psychosis, where the drug triggers a psychotic episode that may persist after the acute intoxication has resolved.[219] Nonetheless, psychotic symptoms in the context of hallucinogen use have been reported, and hallucinogens[220] can trigger psychosis in people with existing psychotic illnesses or a predisposition to psychosis, but also in people with no pre-existing mental health problems.[221]

Effects on Physical Health

Hallucinogen NPS can result in a range of adverse physical effects, including nausea, vomiting,[222] diarrhoea,[223] non-specific gastric discomfort, headache, tachycardia,[224] hypertension, feelings of heat and cold, dizziness, weakness, tremors, drowsiness, paraesthesia, blurred vision, dilated pupils, hyperthermia[225] and hypoglycaemia.[226] Reported musculoskeletal effects include myalgias, twitching, muscle tension and jaw clenching, shaking and increased tendon reflexes.[227] Tachypnoea, metabolic acidosis, rhabdomyolysis and acute kidney injury/acute kidney failure have also been reported.

Individuals may also present with trauma related to accidents resulting from behaviours undertaken while intoxicated.

Traditional hallucinogens – for example, LSD and psilocybin – have low systemic toxicity unless very large doses are ingested.[228] Accidental overdoses are rare with traditional hallucinogens. In contrast, some of the newer hallucinogen NPS have narrower safety ratios, and so carry greater risk of acute toxicity and severe adverse effects.

The patterns of systemic toxicity vary across the hallucinogen NPS and include:

- **Sympathomimetic toxicity:** Some hallucinogen NPS have the potential to cause toxicity with stimulant features. Severe and life-threatening sympathomimetic toxicity has been reported (e.g. Ayahuasca, and 2 C series, NBOMes and bromo-dragonflyα-Methyltryptamine/αMT).[229][210]

- **Serotonin syndrome:** Some hallucinogen NPS cause serotonin syndrome (e.g. 5-MeO-DiPT), particularly when taken in combination with other serotonergic drugs such as MDMA, monoamine oxidase inhibitors or selective serotonin reuptake inhibitor antidepressants.

18.6   Management of Acute Health Harms

There is no antidote available to reverse the effects of hallucinogens. The management of mild to moderate toxicity should be supportive. Individuals should be treated in low-stimulus, brightly lit environments with verbal reassurance. Benzodiazepines may be required to control agitation. In cases of severe intoxication or other complications, transfer to acute medical setting for further monitoring may be required.[230]

18.7   Health Harms from Repeated Use

Considering the powerful psychoactive effects produced by hallucinogen NPS, there is surprisingly little evidence of adverse health consequences from prolonged use. The main reported harm is Hallucinogen Persisting Perception Disorder (HPPD).

18.7.1   Hallucinogen Persisting Perception Disorder (HPPD)

Halpern et al.[231] described Hallucinogen Persisting Perception Disorder (HPPD) as a re-experiencing of some perceptual distortions induced while intoxicated, and suggested that this can cause functional impairment and anxiety. HPPD is associated with classical hallucinogenic drugs, but also with other substances, including natural and synthetic cannabinoids.[232]

HPPD is typically associated with visual disturbances. Tracers, trailing phenomena, after images (palinopsia), haloes around object, intensification of colour, flashing colours, geometric imagery and visual 'snow' appear to be common and resistant symptoms. Other visual symptoms can include teleopsia, pelopsia, macropsia, micropsia and false perception of movement of images in the peripheral field.[233] Dissociative symptoms, including depersonalisation and derealisation, are also consistently associated with HPPD.

Two forms of HPPD have been described:

- **HPPD Type I** or brief flashbacks (also known as Benign Flashback and Flashback Type HPPD). HPPD Type I is short-term, reversible and benign. HPPD I is typically associated with 'auras', minor feelings of self-detachment, mild bewilderment, and mild depersonalisation and derealisation.[234]

- Although it can provoke unpleasant feelings, it is not associated with significant concern, distress or impairment in individual, familial, social, occupational or other important areas of functioning. The impairment is mild and the prognosis is usually good.

- **HPPD Type II** is suggested to have a chronic, relapsing and remitting course, with fluctuating symptoms lasting months or even years. The impairment of HPPD II is severe, with visual distortions and dissociative effects causing significant distress. The prognosis is worse than for HPPD Type 1.[235]

It has been suggested that in most cases HPPD is due to a subtle over-activation of predominantly neural visual pathways after the use of hallucinogens. Factors that may predict vulnerability to HPPD include individual or family histories of anxiety and pre-drug-use complaints of tinnitus, eye floaters and concentration problems.

18.8 Case 12 Hallucinogen Persisting Perception Disorder

Presenting Complaint/History

Adam is a 19-year-old chemistry student living with three flatmates. He has always been fascinated by hallucinogens and first took LSD aged 14. During adolescence he experimented with a number of psychoactive substances, including magic mushrooms, cannabis, amphetamines and ketamine. Once he started university he began buying new hallucinogens online 'out of curiosity'. He now only takes hallucinogens, not using any other drugs or alcohol. Adam has identified a number of websites that sell products labelled as 'research chemicals' with promised hallucinogenic effects. He typically consumes these drugs on his own at home, and over the last six months Adam has taken hallucinogens around once a week.

Three weeks ago, Adam bought and consumed a new hallucinogen with a chemical name he did not recognise. The substance arrived in the post in capsule form. Adam consumed one capsule, but after an hour he felt nothing. Wondering if he had been sold 'a dud', he consumed a second capsule, and half an hour later, when he still did not experience any psychoactive effect, he consumed a third. About two hours after taking the first capsule, Adam began to feel dizzy and nauseous. He began to experience intense visual and auditory distortions and was gripped by fear. These effects continued for the next 12 hours, during which Adam barricaded himself in his room and hid under his bed. Eventually the symptoms resolved and, exhausted, Adam fell asleep.

The next day Adam felt very unwell. The hallucinogenic effects were no longer present but he continued to feel nauseous, although this gradually resolved during the day. That evening he began to recover and left his room to get some food at the local shop. Entering the shop, Adam suddenly began to experience visual distortions. Products on the shop counter began to glow and Adam saw after images when he looked away from objects. Nothing in the shop looked 'real' and Adam felt like he had walked onto a film set in which everything he saw was a prop. That night, every time Adam closed his eyes to sleep, he saw bright visual trails and flashing lights behind his eyelids.

Over the next few weeks, the visual distortions continued. Adam felt that his thinking was impaired, and feelings of derealisation came and went. Adam described a 'brain fog' which he could not shake. He was unable to attend lectures or focus on his studies. He also stopped leaving the house as he found social settings too stimulating. After three weeks of these symptoms and with no improvement, he attended the local drug treatment service to ask for help.

Assessment

At assessment, Adam looked exhausted and explained that the visual distortions were interfering with his day-to-day functioning and causing significant insomnia. He expressed concern that he had 'damaged' his brain and would 'never get better'. There was evidence of significant anxiety focused on the symptoms. There was no evidence of a depressive episode or psychosis.

There were no abnormalities on physical examination; specifically, no neurological abnormalities. Routine bloods were performed, which were all within normal range. A diagnosis of HPPD was made.

Management

A course of cognitive behavioural therapy (CBT) was commenced, focusing on anxiety management. Adam was also cautioned about using any further psychoactive substances.

After one month of treatment, Adam had responded well to the CBT. Although his symptoms continued, he felt more able to cope. He returned to his academic studies but found it hard to concentrate and did poorly in his examinations.

Three months later, Adam's symptoms had continued to improve but were still present. He avoided noisy or brightly lit environments as he found them over-stimulating, but was able to see friends again in quiet settings. He avoided all drugs and continued to engage in CBT.

After one year, Adam only experienced the symptoms of HPPD occasionally, when exposed to triggering environments. He continued to avoid environments which he found over-stimulating but no longer experienced derealisation or 'brain fog'.

Key Learning

HPPD is a poorly understood condition which, despite its name, can be caused by a wide range of psychoactive substances.

Symptoms can be highly distressing and typically include visual distortions, derealisation and subjective cognitive impairment. Anxiety about the symptoms is common and may exacerbate the presentation by causing hypervigilance for symptoms.

Currently there are no recommended evidence-based interventions for HPPD besides abstinence from psychoactive substances. Instead, management should focus on identifying and treating co-existing mental health problems such as anxiety and depression.

18.9 Management of Health Harms from Repeated Use

18.9.1 Management of HPPD

There is no established treatment for HPPD. There have been a number of case reports of successful treatment with neuroleptics, anticonvulsants, benzodiazepines and clonidine, but no randomised controlled trials to date. It has been argued that the multifactorial nature of the disorder, and the prominence of co-morbidities, suggest the need for highly individualised treatment. Abstinence from all psychoactive substances, anxiety management interventions and treatment of co-morbid disorders is suggested.[236]

Concluding Remarks

As this book has illustrated, the illicit drug market is undergoing a period of unprecedented change. This dynamic situation has resulted in a huge number of new psychoactive drugs being available to those who seek them. Prevalence studies suggest that young people, clubbers, students and men who have sex with men are particularly likely to consume emerging drugs, and these groups should be the target for health messages about potential harms. Developing appropriate health messages is a challenge, however, as for many of these emerging drugs, little is known about their psychoactive characteristics and potential to cause health harms.

Clinicians will be understandably concerned by the lack of information and clinical guidance available to assist them in treating those who come to harm. Our suggestion to frontline clinical staff is to try to identify the broad psychoactive category (stimulant, sedative or hallucinogen) and use clinical guidance and protocols available for established drugs in these categories. In doing so, clinicians should be able to formulate initial treatment approaches.

Many emerging drugs have similar health harms to established drugs. Stimulant NPS can cause dangerous cardiotoxicity, while sedative NPS can depress respiratory function. Worryingly, these generalised health harms are often more severe in the emerging drugs, as successive generations are developed to cause greater psychoactive effect.

While many of the health harms of emerging drugs may be generalised to the psychoactive drug group, there are perhaps inevitably unpredictable harms. Urological damage with prolonged ketamine use, severe withdrawals in GHB-dependent people, psychotic symptoms with SCRAs and 'wooden chest' with fentanyl analogues are examples. Careful clinical assessment is critical, and frontline staff will need to be vigilant in the detection of unexpected harms. Early detection and systems to enable rapid sharing of these harms should be considered to assist in developing clinical protocols.

Emerging drugs with poorly understood acute harms and little research to guide treatment will continue to challenge clinicians for the foreseeable future. It is of concern that in most cases the harms from prolonged use remain unknown. Their use appears to be concentrated in younger drug-using populations, a group often considered hard to engage by health services of all types. In many countries, drug treatment services rightly focus their resources on people who use heroin, correctly identifying them as a cohort experiencing great physical and psychiatric harm. Services must challenge the perception of some younger, non-heroin users that drug treatment services are for 'heroin only'. National policy makers and local planners should bear in mind that the number of people experiencing harms from emerging drugs is likely to increase. Responding to this emerging group will require a concerted effort to improve knowledge and understanding of these drugs. This will only be achieved through prioritising research on emerging drugs. As the evidence builds, clinicians will need to develop their skills to feel competent and confident in the management of emerging drug harms. We hope that this book will support clinicians in developing their knowledge, and improve the treatment of people experiencing harms from these new drugs.

References

1. The United Nations Office on Drugs and Crime (UNODC). World Drug Report 2018 (United Nations publication, Sales No. E.18.XI.9). www.unodc.org/wdr2018/ (accessed 2 Jun 2020).
2. The United Nations Office on Drugs and Crime (UNODC). World Drug Report 2019 (United Nations publication, Sales No. E.19.XI.8). https://wdr.unodc.org/ wdr2019/prelaunch/WDR19_Booklet_1_EXECUTIVE_SUMMARY.pdf (accessed 2 April 2020).
3. National Institute of Drug Abuse (NIDA). Club Drugs. www.drugabuse.gov/drugs-abuse/club-drugs (accessed 2 April 2020).
4. The United Nations Office on Drugs and Crime (UNODC). Early Warning Advisory on New Psychoactive Substances. www.unodc.org/LSS/Page/NPS (accessed 2 April 2020).
5. Owie RE, Gosney P, Roney A, O'Brien A. Psychiatrists' knowledge of novel psychoactive substances. *Drugs and Alcohol Today* 2017;17(3):178–85, https://doi.org /10.1108/DAT-03-2017-0011
6. European Monitoring Centre for Drugs and Drug Addiction. *European Drug Report 2019: Trends and Developments*. Luxembourg: Publications Office of the European Union, 2019.
7. Corazza O, Schifano F, Farre M, et al. Designer drugs on the internet: a phenomenon out-of-control? The emergence of hallucinogenic drug Bromo-Dragonfly. *Curr Clin Pharmacol.* 2011 May;6(2):125–9.
8. Measham F, Moore K, Newcombe R, Welch Z. Tweaking, bombing, dabbing and stockpiling: the emergence of mephedrone and the perversity of prohibition. *Drugs Alcohol Today* 2010;10(1):14–21.
9. Measham F, Wood DM, Dargan PI, Moore K. The rise in legal highs: prevalence and patterns in the use of illegal drugs and first- and second-generation 'legal highs' in South London gay dance clubs. *J Substance Use* August 2011;16(4):263–72.
10. Brunt TM, Poortman A, Niesink RJ, van den Brink W. Instability of the ecstasy market and a new kid on the block: mephedrone. *J Psychopharmacol.* 2011 Nov;25 (11):1543–7. doi:10.1177/0269881110378370
11. Home Office. Drug Misuse Declared: Findings from the 2011/12 Crime Survey for England and Wales (2nd Edition) July 2012. https://assets.publishing.service.gov.uk /government/uploads/system/uploads/attachment_data/file/147938/drugs-misuse-dec-1112-pdf.pdf (accessed 1 April 2020)
12. Public Health England. Adult Substance Misuse Statistics from the National Drug Treatment Monitoring System (NDTMS) 1 April 2017 to 31 March 2018. November 2018 PHE publications gateway number: 2018575 https://assets

.publishing.service.gov.uk/government/uploads/system/uploads/attachment_data/file/752993/AdultSubstanceMisuseStatisticsfromNDTMS2017-18.pdf (accessed 1 April 2020)

13. Office of National Statistics. Deaths Related to Drug Poisoning in England and Wales. 2018 Registrations August 2019 www.ons.gov.uk/peoplepopulationand community/birthsdeathsandmarriages/deaths/bulletins/deathsrelatedtodrugpoiso ninginenglandandwales/2018registrations (accessed 2 April 2020)

14. Home Office. Seizures of Drugs in England and Wales, Financial Year Ending 2018 Statistical Bulletin 26/18 November 2018 https://assets.publishing.service.gov.uk/g overnment/uploads/system/uploads/attachment_data/file/754677/seizures-drugs-mar2018-hosb2618.pdf (accessed 2 April 2020).

15. European Monitoring Centre for Drugs and Drug Addiction and Europol. *EU Drug Markets Report: In-Depth Analysis, EMCDDA–Europol Joint publications, 2016* Luxembourg: Publications Office of the European Union.

16. European Monitoring Centre for Drugs and Drug Addiction and Europol. *Drugs and the Darknet: Perspectives for Enforcement, Research and Policy, EMCDDA–Europol Joint publications*, 2017. Luxembourg: Publications Office of the European Union.

17. European Monitoring Centre for Drugs and Drug Addiction EMCDDA. *Recent changes in Europe's cocaine market. Results from an EMCDDA trendspotter study*, 2018. Portugal, Lisbon: European Monitoring Centre for Drugs and Drug Addiction.

18. Clinical Guidelines on Drug Misuse and Dependence Update. *Independent Expert Working Group (2017) Drug misuse and dependence: UK Guidelines on Clinical Management.* London: Department of Health, 2017.

19. World Health Organisation International Classification of Diseases, 11th Revision (ICD-11) Disorders due to Substance Use or Addictive Behaviours https://icd .who.int/browse11/l-m/en#/http%3a%2f%2fid.who.int%2ficd%2fentity%2f160266 9465 (accessed 2 April 2020).

20. National Institute for Health and Clinical Excellence. Drug Misuse: Psychosocial Interventions (Clinical Guideline 51). 2007.

21. National Institute for Health and Clinical Excellence. Drug Misuse in Over 16s: Opioid Detoxification Clinical Guideline. Published 25 July 2007.

22. National Institute for Health and Clinical Excellence. Alcohol Use Disorders: Harmful Drinking and Alcohol Dependence (Clinical Guidance 115: Evidence Update). 2013.

23. National Institute for Health and Clinical Excellence. Behaviour Change: Individual Approaches (PH 49). 2014.

24. Darke S, Kaye S, McKetin R, et al. Major physical and psychological harms of methamphetamine use. *Drug Alcohol Rev* 2008;27:253–62.

25. Pérez-Mañá C, Castells X, Torrens M, Capellà D, Farre M. Efficacy of psychostimulant drugs for amphetamine abuse or dependence (Review). *Cochrane Database Syst Rev.* 2013 Sep. 2;9:CD009695. doi:10.1002/14651858.CD009695. pub2

26. European Monitoring Centre for Drugs and Drug Addiction (EMCDDA). *The Levels of Use of Opioids, Amphetamines and Cocaine and Associated Levels of Harm: Summary of Scientific Evidence.* March 2014.

27. Carvalho M, Carmo H, Costa VM, et al. Toxicity of amphetamines: an update. *Arch Toxicol.* 2012 Aug;86(8):1167–231. doi:10.1007/s00204-012-0815-5

28. Henry JA, Jeffreys KJ, Dawling S. Toxicity and deaths from 3,4-methylenedioxy-methamphetamine ('ecstasy'). *Lancet.* 1992;340:384–7.

29. Green AR, O'Shea E, Colado MI. A review of the mechanisms involved in the acute MDMA (ecstasy)-induced hyperthermic response. *Eur J Pharmacol.* 2004;500 (1–3):3–13.

30. Boyer EW, Shannon M. The serotonin syndrome. *N Engl J Med.* 2005;352:1112–20.

31. Dunkley EJ, Isbister GK, Sibbritt D, Dawson AH, Whyte IM. The Hunter serotonin toxicity criteria: simple and accurate diagnostic decision rules for serotonin toxicity. *QJM.* 2003;96:635–42.

32. Sun-Edelstein C, Tepper SJ, Shapiro RE. Drug-induced serotonin syndrome: a review. *Expert Opin Drug Saf.* 2008 Sep;7(5):587–96. doi:10.1517/14740338.7.5.587

33. Gillman PK. Triptans, serotonin agonists, and serotonin syndrome (serotonin toxicity): a review. *Headache* 2010;50:264–72.

34. Huether G, Zhou D, Ruther E. Causes and consequences of the loss of serotonergic presynapses elicited by the consumption of 3,4-methylenedioxymethamphetamine (MDMA, 'ecstasy') and its congeners. *J Neural Transm.* 1997;104:771–94.

35. Parrott AC. Recreational ecstasy/MDMA, the serotonin syndrome, and serotonergic neurotoxicity. *Pharmacol Biochem Behav.* 2002;71:837–44.

36. Turkel SB, Nadala JG, Wincor MZ. Possible serotonin syndrome in association with 5-HT(3) antagonist agents. *Psychosomatics.* 2001;42:258–60.

37. Isbister GK, Bowe SJ, Dawson A, Whyte IM. Relative toxicity of selective serotonin reuptake inhibitors (SSRIs) in overdose. *J Toxicol Clin Toxicol.* 2004;42:277–85.

38. Home Office. Drugs Misuse: Findings from the 2018/19 Crime Survey for England and Wales Statistical Bulletin: 21/19. 19 September 2019.

39. Bachia K, Manib V, Jeyachandranc D, et al. Vascular disease in cocaine addiction. *Atherosclerosis.* 2017;262:154–62. doi:10.1016/j.atherosclerosis.2017.03.019.

40. Riezzo I, Fiore C, De Carlo D, et al. Side effects of cocaine abuse: multiorgan toxicity and pathological consequences. *Curr Med Chem.* 2012;19(33):5624–46.

41. Henning RJ, Wilson LD, Glauser JM. Cocaine plus ethanol is more cardiotoxic than cocaine or ethanol alone. *Crit Care Med.* 1994;22:1896–1906.

42. Wiener SE, Sutijono D, Moon CH, et al. Patients with detectable cocaethylene are more likely to require intensive care unit admission after trauma. *Am J Emerg Med.* 2010;28:1051.

43. Srisurapanont M, Ali R, Marsden J, et al. Psychotic symptoms in methamphetamine psychotic in-patients. *Int J Neuropsychopharmacol.* 2003;6(4):347–52.

44. Arunogiril S, Foulds JA, McKetin R, Lubman DI. A systematic review of risk factors for methamphetamine-associated psychosis. *Aust N Z J Psychiatry* 2018;52(6):514–29. DOI:10.1177/0004867417748750

45. Arunogiri S, McKetin R, Verdejo-Garcia A, et al. The methamphetamine-associated psychosis spectrum: a clinically focused review. *Int J Ment Health Addiction* 2020;18:54–65. https://doi.org/10.1007/s11469-018-9934-4

46. McKentin R. Methamphetamine psychosis: insights from the past. *Addiction* 2018;113(8):1522–27.

47. Rawson RA, Ling W. Clinical management: methamphetamine. In: Galanter M, Kleber HD, eds. *Textbook of Substance Abuse Treatment*, 2008 4th ed. pp. 169–79. Washington, DC, American Psychiatric Publishing.

48. Akiyama K. Longitudinal clinical course following pharmacological treatment of methamphetamine psychosis which persists after long-term abstinence. *Ann N Y Acad Sci.*2006;1074:125–34.

49. Ma J, Li XD, Wang TY, et al. Relationship between the duration of methamphetamine use and psychotic symptoms: A two-year prospective cohort study *Drug Alcohol Depend.* 2018;187:363–69. doi:10.1016/j.drugalcdep.2018.03.023.

50. Glasner-Edwards S, Mooney LJ, Marinelli-Casey P, et al. Psychopathology in methamphetamine-dependent adults 3 years after treatment. *Drug Alcohol Rev.* 2010;29:12–20.

51. McKetin R, Dawe S, Burns R, et al. The profile of psychiatric symptoms exacerbated by methamphetamine use. *Drug and Alcohol Dependence* 2016;61(1):104–9. http://dx.doi.org/10.1016/j.drugalcdep.2016.01.018

52. Bell DS, Trethowan WH. Amphetamine addiction and disturbed sexuality. *Arch Gen Psychiatry.* 1961;4:74–8.

53. Buchacz K, McFarland W, Kellogg T, et al. Amphetamine use is associated with increased HIV incidence among men who have sex with men in San Francisco. *AIDS.* 2005;19:1423–4.

54. McKetin R, Lubman DI, Baker A, et al. The relationship between methamphetamine use and heterosexual behaviour: evidence from a prospective longitudinal study. *Addiction.* 2018;113(7):1276–85. doi:10.1111/add.14181.

55. Bourne A, Reid D, Hickson F, et al. A perfect storm? Modern technological and structural facilitators of drug use during sex among gay men in London. Poster presentation, 2014. Available from www.sigmaresearch.org.uk/files/Adam_Bourn e_IAS_Melbourne_2014e_poster.pdf.

56. Gilbart VL, Simms I, Jenkins C, et al. Sex, drugs and smart phone applications: findings from semistructured interviews with men who have sex with men diagnosed with Shigella flexneri in England and Wales. *Sex Transm Infect.* 2015;91 (8):598–602. doi:10.1136/sextrans-2015-052014.

57. Hopwood MN, Cama E, Treloar C. *Methamphetamine use among men who have sex with men in Australia: A literature review.* 2016. UNSW Australia: Centre for Social Research in Health.

58. Nichols DE. Differences between the mechanism of action of MDMA, MBDB, and the classic hallucinogens. Identification of a new therapeutic class: entactogens. *J Psychoactive Drugs.* 1986;18:305–13.

59. De la Torre RM. Human pharmacology of MDMA: pharmacokinetics, metabolism, and disposition. *Therapeutic Drug Monitoring.* 2004;26(2):137–44.

60. Feduccia AA, Holland J, Mithoefer MC. Progress and promise for the MDMA drug development program. *Psychopharmacology* 2018;235(2):561–71. doi 10.1007/s00213-017-4779-2.

61. Schenk S, Newcombe D. Methylenedioxymethamphetamine (MDMA) in psychiatry: pros, cons, and suggestions. *J Clin Psychopharmacol* 2018;38(6): 632–38. doi:10.1097/JCP.0000000000000962

62. Home Office. Drug Misuse: Findings from the 2017/18 Crime Survey for England and Wales. *Statistical Bulletin*, 14/18 July 2018.

63. Brunt TM, Poortman A, Niesink RJ, van den Brink W. Instability of the ecstasy market and a new kid on the block: Mephedrone. *J Psychopharmacol*, 2011;25:1543–47.

64. McElrath K, Van Hout MC. A preference for mephedrone: drug markets, drugs of choice, and the emerging 'legal high' scene. *J Drug Issues*. 2011;41 (4):487–507.

65. EMCDDA. European drug report. Trends and developments 2015. Luxembourg: Publications Office of the European Union. 2015. Retrieved from www.emcdda.europa.eu/system/files/publications/2473/TD0116348ENN.pdf

66. Edland-Gryta M, Sandberga S, Pedersen W. From ecstasy to MDMA: Recreational drug use, symbolic boundaries, and drug trends International *Journal of Drug Policy* 50;2017:1–8.

67. European Monitoring Centre for Drugs and Drug Addiction. *Recent changes in Europe's MDMA/ecstasy market, EMCDDA Rapid Communication*. 2016. Luxembourg: Publications Office of the European Union.

68. Public Health Wales. PHILTRE Annual Report 2017–18: www.wales.nhs.uk/sites plus/documents/888/Philtre%20Annual%20Report%202018%20FINAL.pdf (accessed 15 January 2019).

69. Ling LH, Marchant C, Buckley NA, Prior M, Irvine RJ. Poisoning with the recreational drug paramethoxyamphetamine ('death'). *Med J Australia*. 2001;174:453–5.

70. Baylen CA. A review of the acute subjective effects of MDMA/ecstasy. *Addiction*. 2006;101(7):933–47.

71. Green AR, Mechan AO, Elliott JM, O'Shea E, Colado MI. The pharmacology and clinical pharmacology of 3,4-methylenedioxymethamphetamine (MDMA, 'ecstasy'). *Pharmacological Reviews*. 2003;55(3):463–508.

72. Sáez-Briones P, Hernández A. MDMA (3, 4-methylenedioxymethamphetamine) analogues as tools to characterize MDMA-like effects: an approach to understand entactogen pharmacology. *Current Neuropharmacology*. 2013;11(5):521.

73. Degenhardt L, Hall W. *The Health and Psychological Effects of 'Ecstasy' (MDMA) Use. National Drug and Alcohol Research Centre*. University of New South Wales, 2010.

74. Rosenson J, Smollin C, Sporer KA, Blanc P, Olson KR. Patterns of ecstasy-associated hyponatremia in California. *Ann Emerg Med*. 2007;49(2):164–71, 171.e1.

75. Rogers G, Elston J, Garside R, et al. The harmful health effects of recreational ecstasy: a systematic review of observational evidence. *Health Technol Assess*. 2009;13(6):iii–iv, ix–xii. doi:10.3310/hta13050

76. Jahns F-P, Auzinger G, Pineau Mitchell A. Too hot to handle: A case report of extreme pyrexia after MDMA ingestion. *Therapeutic Hypothermia and Temperature Management* 2018;8(3):173–75. doi:10.1089/ther.2018.0002

77. Grunau BE, Wiens MO, Brubacher JR. Dantrolene in the treatment of MDMA-related hyperpyrexia: a systematic review. *CJEM.* 2010;12(5):435–42.

78. Chang JCYC. Late diagnosis of MDMA-related severe hyponatremia. *Case Rep Intern Med.* 2014;1(2):153.

79. Meehan TJ, Bryant SM, Aks SE. Drugs of abuse: the highs and lows of altered mental states in the emergency department. *Emerg Med Clin North Am.* 2010;28(3):663–82. doi:10.1016/j. emc.2010.03.012.

80. Reddy P, Mooradian AD. Diagnosis and management of hyponatraemia in hospitalised patients. *Int J Clin Pract,* 2009;63(10):1494–508. doi:10.1111/j.1742-1241.2009.02103.

81. Parrott AC. Chronic tolerance to recreational MDMA (3,4-methylenedioxymethamphetamine) or ecstasy. *J Psychopharmacol.* 2005;19:71–83.

82. Raznahan M, Hassanzadeh E, Houshmand A, et al. Change in frequency of acute and subacute effects of ecstasy in a group of novice users after 6 months of regular use. *Psychiatr Danub.* 2013;25(2):175–8.

83. Rogers G, Elston J, Garside R, et al. The harmful health effects of recreational ecstasy: a systematic review of observational evidence. *Health Technol Assess.* 2009;13(6):iii–iv, ix–xii. doi:10.3310/hta13050.

84. Hermle L, Spitzer M, Borchardt D, Kovar KA, Gouzoulis E. Psychological effects of MDE in normal subjects. Are entactogens a new class of psychoactive agents? *Neuropsychopharmacology.* 1993;8(2):171–6.

85. Degenhardt L, Bruno R, Topp L. Is ecstasy a drug of dependence? *Drug Alcohol Depend.* 2010;107:1–10.

86. Bruno R, Matthews AJ, Topp L, Degenhardt L, Gomez R, Dunn M. Can the severity of dependence scale be usefully applied to 'ecstasy'? *Neuropsychobiology.* 2009;60 (3–4):137–47. doi:10.1159/000253550

87. Baumann MH, Partilla JS, Lehner KR. Psychoactive 'bath salts': Not so soothing. *European Journal of Pharmacology* 2013;698:1–5. doi:10.1016/j.ejphar.2012.11.020

88. Majchrzak M, Celiński R, Kuś P, et al. The newest cathinone derivatives as designer drugs: an analytical and toxicological review. *Forensic Toxicol* 2018;36:33–50 http s://doi.org/10.1007/s11419-017-0385-6

89. Glennon RA, Dukat M. Synthetic cathinones: a brief overview of overviews with applications to the forensic sciences. *Ann Forensic Res Anal.* 2017;4(2):1040.

90. Daveluy A, Géniaux H, Eiden C, et al. Illicit drugs or medicines taken by parachuting. *Fundamental & Clinical Pharmacology* 2016;30(2):185–190.

91. Ross EA, Reisfield GM, Watson MC, Chronister CW, Goldberger BA. Psychoactive 'bath salts' intoxication with methylenedioxypyrovalerone. *The American Journal of Medicine* 2012;125(9):854–8. doi: 10.1016/j.amjmed.2012.02.019 PMID:22682791

92. Karila L, Billieux J, Benyamina A, Lançon C, Cottencin O, The effects and risks associated to mephedrone and methylone in humans: a review of the preliminary evidences. *Brain Research Bulletin.* 2016;126:61–7.

93. Gatch MB, Forster MJ. Entactogenic effects of synthetic cathinones. *Abstracts/ Drug and Alcohol Dependence* 2017;171:e2–e226.

94. Colon-Perez LM, Tran K, Thompson K, et al. The psychoactive designer drug and bath salt constituent MDPV causes widespread disruption of brain functional connectivity. *Neuropsychopharmacology* 2016;41:2352–65.

95. Homman L, Seglert J, Morgan MJ. An observational study on the sub-acute effects of mephedrone on mood, cognition, sleep and physical problems in regular mephedrone users. *Psychopharmacology* 2018;235(9):2609–18. doi:10.1007/s00213-018-4953-1

96. Wood DM, Davies S, Greene SL, et al. Case series of individuals with analytically confirmed acute mephedrone toxicity. *Clin Toxicol.* 2010;48:924–7.

97. Wood DM, Davies S, Puchnarewicz M, et al. Recreational use of mephedrone (4-methylmethcathinone, 4-MMC) with associated sympathomimetic toxicity. *J Med Toxicol.* 2010;6(3):327–30.

98. Fleckenstein AE, Volz TJ, Riddle EL, Gibb JW, Hanson GR. New insights into the mechanism of action of amphetamines. *Annu Rev Pharmacol Toxicol.* 2007;47:681–98.

99. Dargan PI, Sedefov R, Gallegos A, Wood DM. The pharmacology and toxicology of the synthetic cathinone mephedrone (4-methylmethcathinone). *Drug Test Anal.* 2011;3(7–8):454–63. doi:10.1002/dta.312

100. German CL, Fleckenstein AE, Hanson GR. Bath salts and synthetic cathinones: an emerging designer drug phenomenon. *Life Sci.* 2014;97:2–8.

101. Prosser JM, Nelson LS. The toxicology of bath salts: a review of synthetic cathinones. *J Med Toxicol.* 2012;8:33–42.

102. Woo TM, Hanley J. 'How do they look?' Identification and treatment of common ingestions in adolescents. *J Pediatr Health Care.* 2013;27(2):135–44. doi:10.1016/j.pedhc.2012.12.002.

103. Simmler LD, Buser TA, Donzelli M, et al. *Pharmacological characterization of designer cathinones in vitro. British Journal of Pharmacology* 2013;168:458–470.

104. EMCDDA. Technical Report on 1-(1,3-benzodioxol-5-yl)-2-(pyrrolidin-1-yl)pentan-1-one (3,4-methylenedioxypyrovalerone, MDPV) Annex 2. Prepared by Ms Alison M Dines, Dr David M Wood and Dr Paul I Dargan: www.emcdda.europa.eu/attachements.cfm/att_228256_EN_TDAK14003ENN.pdf

105. Advisory Council on the Misuse of Drugs (ACMD). *Consideration of the Cathinones.* Home Office, 2010.

106. Winstock A, Mitcheson L, Ramsey J, et al. Mephedrone: use, subjective effects and health risks. *Addiction.* 2011;106(11):1991–6.

107. EMCDDA. Report on the risk assessment of mephedrone in the framework of the Council Decision on new psychoactive substances 2011. www.emcdda.europa.eu/system/files/publications/571/TDAK11001ENC_WEB-OPTIMISED_FILE_280269.pdf

108. EMCDDA. *Risk assessment report of a new psychoactive substance: 4-methylmethcathinone (mephedrone). In accordance with Article 6 of Council Decision 2005/387/JHA on information exchange, risk assessment and control of new psychoactive*

substances.2010. www.emcdda.europa.eu/attachements.cfm/att_116485_EN_Risk%20Assessment%20Report%20on%20mephedrone.pdf

109. Hope VD, Cullen KJ, Smith J, et al. 2016. Is the recent emergence of mephedrone injecting in the United Kingdom associated with elevated risk behaviours and blood borne virus infection? *Eurosurveillance*, 21(19). doi:10.2807/1560-7917.ES.2016.21.19.30225

110. Maitre M. The gamma-hydroxybutyrate signalling system in brain: organization and functional implications. *Prog Neurobiol*. 1997;51:337–61.

111. Schep LJ, Knudsen K, Slaughter RJ, Vale JA, Mégarbane B. The clinical toxicology of γ-hydroxybutyrate, γ-butyrolactone and 1,4-butanediol. *Clin Toxicol (Phila)*. 2012;50(6):458–70. doi:10.3109/15563650.2012.7022

112. Yanagihara Y, Kariya S, Ohtani M, et al. Involvement of CYP2B6 in n-demethylation of ketamine in human liver microsomes. *Drug Metab Dispos*. 2001;29:887–90.

113. European Monitoring Centre for Drugs and Drug Addiction (EMCDDA). Report on the Risk Assessment of GHB in the Framework of the Joint Action on New Synthetic Drugs. 2002. www.emcdda.europa.eu/system/files/publications/175/Risk4_62945.pdf

114. Carter LP, Chen W, Wu H, et al. Comparison of the behavioral effects of gamma-hydroxybutyric acid (GHB) and its 4-methyl-substituted analog, gamma-hydroxyvaleric acid (GHV). *Drug and Alcohol Dependence* 2005;78(1):91–9 https://doi.org/10.1016/j.drugalcdep.2004.10.002

115. Miróa Ò, Galiciaa M, Darganb P, et al. Euro-DEN Research Group: Intoxication by gamma hydroxybutyrate and related analogues: Clinical characteristics and comparison between pure intoxication and that combined with other substances of abuse. *Toxicology Letters* 2017;277:84–91 https://doi.org/10.1016/j.toxlet.2017.05.030

116. Degenhardt L, Darke S, Dillon P. GHB use among Australians: characteristics, use patterns and associated harm. *Drug Alcohol Depend*. 2002;67(1):89–94.

117. Chin RL, Sporer KA, Cullison B, Dyer JE, Wu TD. Clinical course of gamma-hydroxybutyrate overdose. *Ann Emerg Med*. 1998;31(6):716–22.

118. TOXBASE. www.toxbase.org/Chemical-incidents/Management-Pages/GHB-overdose–features-and-management1/ (accessed 16 January 2019).

119. Reeves J, Duda R. GHB/GBl intoxication and withdrawal: a review and case presentation. *Addict Disord Treatment*. 2003;2:25–8.

120. McDonough M, Kennedy N, Glasper A, Bearn J. Clinical features and management of gammahydroxybutyrate (GHB) withdrawal: a review. *Drug Alcohol Depend*. 2004;75:3–9.

121. van Noorden MS, Mol T, Wisselink J, Kuijpers W, Dijkstra BA. Treatment consumption and treatment re-enrollment in GHB-dependent patients in The Netherlands. *Drug and Alcohol Dependence*. 2017;176:96–101.

122. Bell J, Collins R. Gamma-butyrolactone (GBL) dependence and withdrawal. *Addiction*. 2011;106(2):442–7. doi:10.1111/j.1360-0443.2010.03145.x.

123. Lingford-Hughes A, Patel Y, Bowden-Jones O, et al. Improving GHB withdrawal with baclofen: study protocol for a feasibility study for a randomised controlled trial. *Trials* 2016;17:472. https://doi.org/10.1186/s13063-016-1593-9

124. Harmen B, Kamal RM, de Jong CAJ, Dijkstra BAG, Arnt FAS. Baclofen to prevent pelapse in Gamma-Hydroxybutyrate (GHB)-dependent patients: a multicentre, open-label, nonrandomized, controlled trial. *CNS Drugs* 2018;32:437–42 https://doi.org/10.1007/s40263-018-0516-6

125. Dijkstra BAG, Kamal RM, van Noordena MS, et al. Detoxification with titration and tapering in gamma-hydroxybutyrate (GHB) dependent patients: The Dutch GHB monitor project. *Drug and Alcohol Dependence* 2017:170164–173 http://dx.doi.org/10.1016/j.drugalcdep.2016.11.014

126. Pereira FR, McMaster M, van den Brink W, van Wingen G. Effects of gamma hydroxybutyrate (GHB) induced coma on long-term memory and brain function. *Amsterdam Neuroscience*: www.ecnp.eu/presentationpdfs/71/P.6.d.006.pdf (accessed 6 April 2020).

127. UNODC. Fentanyl and its analogues – 50 years on. *Global SMART Update*. 2017;17: www.unodc.org/documents/scientific/Global_SMART_Update_17_web.pdf (accessed 23 March 2020).

128. UNODC. Understanding the global opioid crisis. *Global SMART Update*. 2019;21: www.unodc.org/documents/scientific/Global_SMART_21_web_new.pdf (accessed 27 March 2020).

129. Ayres WA, Starsiak MJ, Sokolay P. The bogus drug: three methyl and alpha methyl fentanyl sold as 'China White'. *J Psychoactive Drugs* 1981;13(1):91–3.

130. Pearson J, Poklis J, Poklis A, et al. Postmortem toxicology findings of acetyl fentanyl, fentanyl, and morphine in heroin fatalities in Tampa, Florida. *Acad Forensic Pathol*. 2015;5(4):676–89.

131. European Monitoring Centre for Drugs and Drug Addiction. European Drug Report 2017: Trends and Developments. 2017. Luxembourg: Publications Office of the European Union.

132. Frank RG, Pollack HA. Addressing the fentanyl threat to public health. *N Engl J Med* 2017;376(7):605–7. doi:10.1056/NEJMp1615145

133. Suzuki J, El-Haddad S. A review: fentanyl and non-pharmaceutical fentanyls. *Drug Alcohol Depend*. 2016;171:107–16. doi:10.1016/j.drugalcdep.2016.11.033

134. European Monitoring Centre for Drugs and Drug Addiction. *Report on the Risk Assessment of Nphenyl-N-[1-(2-phenylethyl)piperidin-4-yl]furan-2-carboxamide (Furanylfentanyl) in the Framework of the Council Decision on New Psychoactive Substances*. December 2017. Lisbon: EMCDDA.

135. Higashikawa Y, Suzuki S. Studies on 1-(2-phenethyl)-4-(N-propionylanilino) piperidine (fentanyl) and its related compounds. VI. Structure–analgesic activity relationship for fentanyl, methylsubstituted fentanyls and other analogues. *Forensic Toxicol*. 2008;26(1):1–5. doi:10.1007/s11419-007-0039-1

136. Darke S, Duflou J. The toxicology of heroin-related death: estimating survival times. *Addiction* 2016;111(9):1607–13. doi:10.1111/add.13429

137. Karinen R, Tuv SS, Rogde S, et al. Lethal poisonings with AH-7921 in combination with other substances. *Forensic Sci Int*. 2014;244:e21–e24.

138. Armenian P, Olson A, Anaya A, et al. Fentanyl and a novel synthetic opioid U-47700 masquerading as street 'Norco' in Central California: a case report. *Ann Emerg Med*. 2017;69:87–90.

139. Papsun D, Krywanczyk A, Vose JC, et al. Analysis of MT-45, a novel synthetic opioid, in human whole blood by LC–MS-MS and its identification in a drug-related death. *J Anal Toxicol.* 2016;40(4):313–17. doi:10.1093/jat/bkw012

140. Katselou M, Papoutsis I, Nikolaou P, Spiliopoulou C, Athanaselis S. 2015. AH-7921: the list of new psychoactive opioids is expanded. *Forensic toxicology,* 33 (2):195–201.

141. Coppola M, Mondola R. AH-7921: from potential analgesic medicine to recreational drug. *Int J High Risk Behav Addict.* 2017;6(2):e22593. doi:10.5812/ijhrba.22593

142. Kronstrand R, Thelander G, Lindstedt D, Roman M, Kugelberg FC. Fatal intoxications associated with the designer opioid AH-7921. *Journal of Analytical Toxicology,* 2014;38(8):604.

143. EMCDDA. Technical report on 3,4-dichloro-N-{[1- (dimethylamino)cyclohexyl] methyl}benzamide (AH-7921), EMCDDA, Lisbon, April 2014. www.emcdda.europa.eu/system/files/publications/774/TDAK14002ENN_480892.pdf

144. Elliott S, Brandt S, Smith C. The first reported fatality associated with the synthetic opioid 3,4-dichloro-N-[2-(dimethylamino)cyclohexyl]-Nmethylbenzamide (U-47700) and implications for forensic analysis. *Drug Testing and Analysis* 8(8): 875–9. http://dx.doi.org/10.1002/dta.1984

145. Helander A, Bäckberg M, Beck O. MT-45, a new psychoactive substance associated with hearing loss and unconsciousness. *Clin Toxicol.* 2014;52(8):901–4.

146. Kjellgren A, Jacobsson K, Soussan C. The quest for well-being and pleasure: experiences of the novel synthetic opioids AH-7921 and MT-45, as reported by anonymous users online. *J Addict Res Ther.*2016;7(287):2.

147. Coppola M, Mondola R. MT-45: a new, dangerous legal high. *J Opioid Management* 2014;10:301–2.

148. Siddiqi S, Verney C, Dargan P, et al. Understanding the availability, prevalence of use, desired effects, acute toxicity and dependence potential of the novel opioid MT-45. *Clin Toxicol.* 2015;53(1):54–9.

149. Mohr ALA, Friscia M, Papsun D, et al. Analysis of novel synthetic opioids U-47700, U-50488 and furanyl fentanyl by LC–MS/MS in postmortem casework. *J Anal Toxicol.* 2016;40:709–17. doi:10.1093/jat/bkw086.

150. Elliott S, Brandt S, Smith C. The first reported fatality associated with the synthetic opioid 3,4-dichloro-N-[2-(dimethylamino)cyclohexyl]-Nmethylbenzamide (U-47700) and implications for forensic analysis. *Drug Testing and Analysis* 2016;8 (8):875–9. http://dx.doi.org/10.1002/dta.1984

151. Public Health England. Guidance for local areas on planning to deal with fentanyl or another potent opioid. 8 May 2018 www.gov.uk/government/publications/fentanyl-preparing-for-a-future-threat/guidance-for-local-areas-on-planning-to-deal-with-fentanyl-or-another-potent-opioid

152. Fairbairn N, Coffin PO, Walley AY. Naloxone for heroin, prescription opioid, and illicitly made fentanyl overdoses: challenges and innovations responding to a dynamic epidemic. *Int J Drug Policy* 2017;46:172–9. doi:10.1016/j.drugpo.2017.06.005

153. Allan J, Herridge N, Griffiths P, et al. Illicit fentanyl use in rural Australia – an exploratory study. *J Alcohol Drug Depend* 2015;3:196. doi:10.4172/23296488.1000196

154. Clinical Guidelines on Drug Misuse and Dependence Update. *Independent Expert Working Group (2017) Drug misuse and dependence: UK guidelines on clinical management.* 2017. London: Department of Health.

155. National Institute for Health and Care Excellence (NICE). Drug misuse in over 16s: opioid detoxification. Clinical guideline: 25 July 2007. www.nice.org.uk/guidance/cg52

156. Arens, AM, Xander MD, van Wijk, MR, et al. Research letter: adverse effects from counterfeit alprazolam tablets. *JAMA Internal Medicine* 2016 176(10):1554–5.

157. Green, TC, Gilbert, M. Counterfeit medications and fentanyl. *JAMA Intern Med.* 2016;176(10):1555–7. doi:10.1001/jamainternmed.2016.4310

158. European Monitoring Centre for Drugs and Drug Addiction. *Fentanils and synthetic cannabinoids: driving greater complexity into the drug situation. An update from the EU Early Warning System (June 2018).* 2018. Luxembourg: Publications Office of the European Union.

159. Łukasik-Głębocka M, Sommerfeld K, Teżyk A, et al. Flubromazolam – a new life-threatening designer benzodiazepine. *Clin Toxicol (Phila).* 2016;54(1):66–8. doi:10.3109/15563650.2015.1112907.

160. Berman RM, Cappiello A, Anand A, et al. Antidepressant effects of ketamine in depressed patients. *Biol Psychiatry.* 2000;47(4):351–4.

161. Singh I, Morgan C, Curran V, et al. Ketamine treatment for depression: opportunities for clinical innovation and ethical foresight. *The Lancet Psychiatry* 2017;4 (5):419–26.

162. Corazza O, Schifano F, Simonato P, et al. Phenomenon of new drugs on the internet: the case of ketamine derivative methoxetamine. *Hum Psychopharmacol.* 2012;27(2):145–9. doi:10.1002/hup.1242.

163. Teltzrow R, Bosch OG. Ecstatic anaesthesia: ketamine and GHB between medical use and selfexperimentation. *Applied Cardiopulmonary Pathophysiology.* 2012;16:309–21.

164. Ross S. Ketamine and addiction. *Primary Psychiatry.* 2008;15(9):61–9.

165. Corazza O, Assi S, Schifano F. From 'Special K' to 'Special M': the evolution of the recreational use of ketamine and methoxetamine. *CNS Neurosci. Ther.* 2013;19 (6):454–60. http://dx.doi.org/10.1111/cns.12063.

166. Siegel RK. Phencyclidine and ketamine intoxication: a study of four populations of recreational users. In: Peterson RC, Stillman RC, eds. *Phencyclidine Abuse: An Appraisal (NIDA Research Monograph 21),* 1978. pp. 119–47. National Institute on Drug Abuse.

167. Morgan CJ, Curran HV. Acute and chronic effects of ketamine upon human memory: a review. *Psychopharmacology (Berl).* 2006;188:408–24.

168. Morgan CJA, Curran HV. Ketamine use: a review. *Addiction.* 2011;107:27–38.

169. Kalsi SS, Wood DM, Dargan PI. The epidemiology and patterns of acute and chronic toxicity associated with recreational ketamine use. *Emerg Health Threats J.* 2011;4:7107. doi:10.3402/ehtj.v4i0.7107.

170. Wood DM, Nicolaou M, Dargan PI. Epidemiology of recreational drug toxicity in a nightclub environment. *Subst Use Misuse.* 2009;44:1495–502.

171. Weiner AL, Vieira L, McKay CA, Bayer MJ. Ketamine abusers presenting to the emergency department: a case series. *J Emerg Med.* 2000;18:447–51.

172. Ng SH, Tse ML, Ng HW, Lau FL. Emergency department presentation of ketamine abusers in Hong Kong: a review of 233 cases. *Hong Kong Med J.* 2010;16(1):6–11.

173. Morgan CJ, Muetzelfeldt L, Curran HV. Consequences of chronic ketamine self-administration upon neurocognitive function and psychological wellbeing: a 1-year longitudinal study. *Addiction.* 2010;105:121–33.

174. Stewart CE. Ketamine as a street drug. *Emerg Med Serv.* 2001;30(11):30, 32, 34 passim.

175. Byer DE, Gould JtAB. Development of tolerance to ketamine in an infant undergoing repeated anesthesia. *Anesthesiology.* 1981;54:255–6.

176. Moore NN, Bostwick JM. Ketamine dependence in anesthesia providers. *Psychosomatics.* 1999;40:356–9.

177. Critchlow DG. A case of ketamine dependence with discontinuation symptoms. *Addiction.* 2006;101(8):1212–13.

178. Lim DK. Ketamine associated psychedelic effects and dependence. *Singapore Med J.* 2003;44:31–4.

179. Wood D. Ketamine and damage to the urinary tract. *Addiction.* 2013;108:1515–19.

180. Wood D, Cottrell A, Baker SC, et al. Recreational ketamine: from pleasure to pain. *BJU Int.* 2011;107(12):1881–4. doi:10.1111/j.1464-410X.2010.10031.x

181. Yew DT, Wood DM, Liang W, Tang HC, Dargan PI. An animal model demonstrating significant bladder inflammation and fibrosis associated with chronic methoxetamine administration. *Clin Toxicol.* 2013;51(4):278.

182. Muetzelfeldt L, Kamboj SK, Rees H, et al. Journey through the K-hole: phenomenological aspects of ketamine use. *Drug Alcohol Depend.* 2008;95(3):219–29. doi:10.1016/j.drugalcdep.2008.01.024

183. Cottrell AM, Gillat DA. Ketamine-associated urinary pathology: the tip of the iceberg for urologists? *British J Med Surg Urol.* 2008;1:136–8.

184. Murray RM, Quigley H, Quattrone D, Englund A, Di Forti M. Traditional marijuana, high-potency cannabis and synthetic cannabinoids: increasing risk for psychosis. *World Psychiatry* 2016;15:195–204.

185. Bonaccorso S, Metastasio A, Ricciardi A, et al. Synthetic cannabinoid use in a case series of patients with psychosis presenting to acute psychiatric settings: clinical presentation and management issues. *Brain Sci.* 2018;8(7):133. doi:10.3390/brainsci8070133

186. Bäckberg M, Tworek L, Beck O, Helander JA. Analytically confirmed intoxications involving MDMB-CHMICA from the STRIDA project. *Med. Toxicol.* 2017;13:52–60. doi:10.1007/s13181-016-0584-2

187. Barceló B, Pichini S, López-Corominas V, et al. Acute intoxication caused by synthetic cannabinoids 5F-ADB and MMB-2201: A case series. *Forensic Science International* 2017;273:e10–e14.

188. EMCDDA. Perspectives on drugs: Synthetic cannabinoids in Europe. www .emcdda.europa.eu/system/files/publications/2753/POD_Synthetic%20cannabi noids_0.pdf

189. Winstock AR, Barratt MJ. Synthetic cannabis: a comparison of patterns of use and effect profile with natural cannabis in a large global sample. *Drug Alcohol Depend.* 2013;131(1–3):106–11. doi:10.1016/j. drugalcdep.2012.12.011

190. Shafi A, Gallagher P, Stewart N, Martinotti G, Corazza O. The risk of violence associated with novel psychoactive substance misuse in patients presenting to acute mental health services. *Hum. Psychopharmacol.* 2017;32:3.

191. Zarifi C, Vyas S. Spice-y kidney failure: A case report and systematic review of acute kidney injury attributable to the use of synthetic cannabis. *Perm J* 2017;21:16–160. https://doi.org/10.7812/TPP/16-160.

192. Nia AB, Medrano B, Perkel C, Galynker I, Hurd YL. Psychiatric comorbidity associated with synthetic cannabinoid use compared to cannabis *Journal of Psychopharmacology* 2016;30(12):1321–30. doi:10.1177/0269881116658990

193. van Amsterdam J, Brunt T, van den Brink W. The adverse health effects of synthetic cannabinoids with emphasis on psychosis-like effects. *Journal of Psychopharmacology* 2015;29(3):254–63.

194. Castellanos D, Thornton G. Synthetic cannabinoid use: recognition and management. *J Psychiatr Pract.* 2012;18(2):86–93. doi:10.1097/01.pra.0000413274.09305.9c.

195. Simmons JR, Skinner CG, Williams J, et al. Intoxication from smoking 'Spice'. *Ann Emerg Med.* 2011;57:187–8.

196. Hurst D, Loeffler G, McLay R. Psychosis associated with synthetic cannabinoid agonists: a case series. *Am J Psychiatry.* 2011;168(10):1119. doi:10.1176/appi. ajp.2011.1101017.https://ajp.psychiatryonline.org/doi/pdf/10.1176/appi.ajp.201 1.11010176

197. Macfarlane V, Christie G. Synthetic cannabinoid withdrawal: a new demand on detoxification services. *Drug and Alcohol Review* 2015;34(2):147–53.

198. European Monitoring Centre for Drugs and Drug Addiction. *New psychoactive substances in prison, EMCDDA Rapid Communication.* 2018. Luxembourg: Publications Office of the European Union.

199. National Offender Management Service. North West 'Through the gate substance misuse services' drug testing project. 2015. www.lgcgroup.com/media/1795/nom s-final-phm-report-version-5.pdf.

200. Blackman S, Bradley, R. From niche to stigma – headshops to prison: exploring the rise and fall of synthetic cannabinoid use among young adults. *International Journal of Drug Policy* 2017;40:70–7.

201. Ralphs R, Williams L, Askey R, Norton A. Adding spice to the porridge: the development of a synthetic cannabinoid market in an English prison. *International Journal of Drug Policy* 2017;40:57–69.

202. Carhart-Harris RL, Goodwin GM. The therapeutic potential of psychedelic drugs: past, present, and future. *Neuropsychopharmacology* 2017;42:2105–113.

203. Garcia-Romeu A, Kersgaard B, Addy PH. Clinical applications of hallucinogens: A review. *Exp Clin Psychopharmacol* 2016;24: 229–68.

204. Bogenschutz MP, Forcehimes AA, Pommy JA, et al. Psilocybin-assisted treatment for alcohol dependence: A proof-of-concept study. *J Psychopharmacol* 2015;29:289–99.

205. Johnson MW, Garcia-Romeu A, Griffiths RR. Long-term follow-up of psilocybin-facilitated smoking cessation. *Am J Drug Alcohol Abuse* 2017;43:55–60.

206. Griffiths RR, Johnson MW, Carducci MA, et al. Psilocybin produces substantial and sustained decreases in depression and anxiety in patients with life-threatening cancer: A randomized double-blind trial. *J Psychopharmacol* 2016;30:1181–97.

207. Byock I. Taking psychedelics seriously. *Journal Of Palliative Medicine* (special report). 2018;21(4).

208. Gee P, Schep LJ, Jensen BP, Moore G, Barrington S. Case series: toxicity from 25B-NBOMe – a cluster of N-bomb cases. *Clinical Toxicology* 2016;54(2):141–6.

209. Timmermann C, Roseman L, Williams L, et al. DMT models the near-death experience. *Frontiers in Psychology* 2018;9:1424.

210. Papoutsis I, Nikolaou P, Stefanidou M, Spiliopoulou C, Athanaselis S. 25B-NBOMe and its precursor 2C-B: modern trends and hidden dangers. *Forensic Toxicol.* 2015;33:1–11. doi:10.1007/s11419-014-0242-9

211. Deluca P, Corazza O, Schifano F, et al. Bromo-dragonfly report. Psychonaut Web-Mapping Project, 2010. www.psychonautproject.eu/documents/reports/Bromodr agonfly.pdf

212. Strassman R. Human psychopharmacology of LSD, dimethyltryptamine and related compounds. In: Pletscher A, Ladewig D, eds. *Fifty Years of LSD: Current Status and Perspectives of Hallucinogens*, pp. 145–74. New York: Parthenon, 1994.

213. Johnstad PG. Powerful substances in tiny amounts: An interview study of psyche-delic microdosing. *Nordic Studies on Alcohol and Drugs* 2018;35(1):39–51.

214. Savulich G, Piercy T, Bruhl AB, et al. Focusing the neuroscience and societal implications of cognitive enhancers. *Clin Pharmacol Ther.* 2017;101(2): 170–2.

215. d'Angelo L-SC, Savulich G, Sahakian BJ. Lifestyle use of drugs by healthy people for enhancing cognition, creativity, motivation and pleasure. *British Journal of Pharmacology.* 2017;174:3257–67.

216. Twemlow SW, Bowen WT. Psychedelic drug-induced psychological crises: atti-tudes of the 'crisis therapist'. *J Psychoactive Drugs.* 1979;11(4):331–5.

217. Johnson M, Richards W, Griffiths R. Human hallucinogen research: guidelines for safety. *J Psychopharmacol.* 2008;22(6):603–20. doi:10.1177/0269881108093587.

218. Reich P, Hepps RB. Homicide during a psychosis induced by LSD. *JAMA.* 1972;219(7):869–71.

219. Keshavan MS, Kaneko Y. Secondary psychoses: an update. *World Psychiatry.* 2013;12(1):4–15.

220. Miyajima M, Matsumoto T, Ito S. 2C-T-4 intoxication: acute psychosis caused by a designer drug. *Psychiatry Clin Neurosci.* 2008;62(2):243.

221. Matsumoto T, Okada T. Designer drugs as a cause of homicide. *Addiction.* 2006;101(11):1666–7.

222. Krebs TS, Johansen P-Ø. Lysergic acid diethylamide (LSD) for alcoholism: meta-analysis of randomized controlled trials. *J Psychopharmacol.* 2012;26 (7):994–1002.

223. Gable RS. Risk assessment of ritual use of oral dimethyltryptamine (DMT) and harmala alkaloids. *Addiction.* 2007;102(1):24–34.

224. Malleson N. Acute adverse reactions to LSD in clinical and experimental use in the United Kingdom. *Br J Psychiatry.* 1971;118(543):229–30.

225. Meehan TJ, Bryant SM, Aks SE. Drugs of abuse: the highs and lows of altered mental states in the emergency department. *Emerg Med Clin North Am.* 2010;28 (3):663–82. doi:10.1016/j. emc.2010.03.012.

226. Boland DM, Andollo W, Hime GW, Hearn WL. Fatality due to acute α-methyltryptamine intoxication. *J Analytic Toxicol.* 2005;29(5):394–7.

227. Alatrash G, Majhail NS, Pile JC. Rhabdomyolysis after ingestion of 'foxy', a hallucinogenic tryptaminederivative. *Mayo Clin Proc.* 2006;81(4):550–1.

228. Gable RS. Comparison of acute lethal toxicity of commonly abused psychoactive substances. *Addiction.* 2004;99(6):686–96.

229. Boland DM, Andollo W, Hime GW, Hearn WL. Fatality due to acute α-methyltryptamine intoxication. *J Analytic Toxicol.* 2005;29(5):394–7.

230. Gee P, Schep LJ, Jensen BP, Moore G, Barrington S. Case series: toxicity from 25B-NBOMe – a cluster of N-bomb cases. *Clinical Toxicology* 2016;54(2)141–6. doi:10.3109/15563650.2015.1115056

231. Halpern JH, Lerner AG, Passie T. A review of hallucinogen persisting perception disorder (HPPD) and an exploratory study of subjects claiming symptoms of HPPD. In Halberstadt AL, Vollenweider FX, Nichols DE (eds), *Behavioral Neurobiology of Psychedelic Drugs. Current Topics in Behavioral Neurosciences,* vol. 36. 2016. Berlin, Heidelberg: Springer.

232. Martinotti G, Santacroce R, Pettorruso M, et al. Hallucinogen persisting perception disorder: etiology, clinical features, and therapeutic perspectives. *Brain Sci.* 2018;8:47. doi:10.3390/brainsci8030047

233. Orsolini L, Papanti GD, De Berardis D, et al. The "endless Trip" among the NPS users: psychopathology and psychopharmacology in the hallucinogen-persisting perception disorder. A systematic review. *Frontiers in Psychiatry.* 2017;8:240. doi:10.3389/fpsyt.2017.00240

234. Lerner AG, Gelkopf M, Skladman I, Oyffe I. Flashback and hallucinogen persisting perception disorder: Clinical aspects and pharmacological treatment approach. *Isr. J. Psychiatry Relat. Sci.* 2002;39:92–99.

235. Halpern JH, Pope Jr HG. Hallucinogen persisting perception disorder: what do we know after 50 years? *Drug Alcohol Depend.* 2003;69:109/119.

236. Hermle L, Simon M, Ruchsow M, Batra A, Geppert M. Hallucinogen persisting perception disorder (HPPD) and flashback – are they identical? *J Alcoholism Drug Depend.* 2013;1:121. doi:10.4172/ jaldd.1000121.

Index

For EU product safety concerns, contact us at Calle de José Abascal, 56–1°,
28003 Madrid, Spain or eugpsr@cambridge.org.

www.ingramcontent.com/pod-product-compliance
Ingram Content Group UK Ltd.
Pitfield, Milton Keynes, MK11 3LW, UK
UKHW040944090126

466816UK00019B/280

Reader's Guides

SECOND SERIES 10

———◦———

MUSIC AND MUSICIANS

by

ALEC ROBERTSON

PUBLISHED FOR
THE NATIONAL BOOK LEAGUE
AT THE UNIVERSITY PRESS
CAMBRIDGE
1956

CAMBRIDGE UNIVERSITY PRESS
Cambridge, New York, Melbourne, Madrid, Cape Town,
Singapore, São Paulo, Delhi, Mexico City

Cambridge University Press
The Edinburgh Building, Cambridge CB2 8RU, UK

Published in the United States of America by Cambridge University Press, New York

www.cambridge.org
Information on this title: www.cambridge.org/9781107622234

First published 1956
Re-issued 2013

A catalogue record for this publication is available from the British Library

ISBN 978-1-107-62223-4 Paperback

CONTENTS

INTRODUCTION

Anyone who broadcasts is liable to receive letters, from listeners unknown to him, which are either congratulatory, critical or downright silly: and without putting it in the category to which, in my opinion, it belongs a sentence from such a letter, which I once received after a talk on music, will serve very well as text for the start of this essay. 'Do not talk to me about music', it began, 'I like it to flow over me in a beautiful golden stream'. The temptation to address the writer, in replying, as 'Dear Mr. Suet Pudding' was almost irresistible; and only for courtesy's sake resisted.

Such a flabby attitude towards the most spiritual of the arts is no doubt the result of regarding music as being primarily, or wholly, a purveyor of emotion and devoid of meaning: a pleasant device to titillate the nerves and play upon the emotions of the listener, or to provide a background against which he can dream dreams or wallow in romantic episodes of his life, past or present. Little wonder, therefore, that the range of music that appeals to such a listener—if he can be said to listen, in any true sense, at all—is small: the 'beautiful golden stream' does not flow into a larger sea. The very type of such a sentimental listener is perhaps Orsino, Duke of Illyria, who opens *Twelfth Night* with the words 'If music be the food of love, play on'; he is obviously a man seeking only for soothing syrup and not for the food that nourishes and strengthens the spiritual part of man.

It was in this sense that Bach is reported to have said that the aim and final reason of all music is the glory of God and the refreshment of the spirit, and that William Blake spoke of music, poetry and painting as 'Man's ways of conversing with Paradise'. Such definitions, also, can be comprehensive enough to include those kinds of music that are a delightful decoration on life and sensibly add to the gaiety of nations.

It may be remembered that when Brahms heard *The Blue Danube* waltz at a party, he wrote a few of the opening bars on the fan of Madame Johann Strauss and put underneath them the words 'unfortunately not by yours truly Johannes Brahms.'

It may be obvious enough, but it needs to be said repeatedly, that music is a communication from the mind and heart and soul of the composer to the listener, made in its own language—which has few analogies with that of any other art and most of those misleading—and delivered, as it has to be, through human channels.

The composer, like all of us, has his full share of human frailties but is marked out from other men by his special gift of expressing himself creatively in musical sounds, and if our education in the arts was more liberal everyone would be able to read the composer's language, and not only those who sing and play.

Bernard Shaw, in this context, remarks in *Music in London* 'people refuse to learn their notes because they feel they will never be able to play well enough to be worth listening to. They might just as well refuse to learn to read because they will never be able to recite or declaim the contents of volumes of poetry well enough to delight an audience'.

It is true that familiarity with the ordinary ways of the musical language undoubtedly develops with constant and appreciative listening: but it has yet to be realised by many sincere lovers of music that great as is its emotional appeal, the emotion is conveyed to us by an exact and calculated process of musical thought. That musical thought ranges from the trivial to the sublime and can even be represented by a unit as small as a couple of notes. The essential thought in the first movement of Beethoven's Fifth Symphony, for example, is conveyed in a phrase of four notes which anybody could have invented, but which only a great master could make the basis of a symphonic movement and subject to such amazing developments.

In this matter of listening to music there must be, of course, no compulsion and the ordinary music lover is certainly not required to bring a trained and analytical ear upon what he hears, but to whatever degree of knowledge he attains he will find his enjoyment thereby deepened, not hindered; and that, as a moment's thought will show, is true of all spheres of knowledge.

Attendances at concerts, attention to broadcasts of 'good' music, and talks on it, the extraordinary sales of long-playing records, all go to prove that an increasingly intelligent interest is being taken in the art, but—and this long preamble is at length reaching its goal—decidedly less interest is taken in books about music.

The idea that the buying of books of any kind is a luxury dies hard, and perhaps the idea of buying a book on music may seem to some an outrageous extravagance; or it may be feared that such books will be full of musical jargon and technical terms, and so prove unintelligible to the 'ordinary' listener; or merely that he may simply be unaware of the large range of such books which he might enjoy, profit from, and want to own. Hence the reason for the Guide that follows: and it would be pleasant and rewarding if it helped to eliminate a cliché one has come to dread. 'I love music but'—here it comes!—'I'm afraid I don't know anything about it'. To which the correct answer is 'why not?' and a copy of this pamphlet.

Most of us develop a strongly marked preference for the work of one composer or, preferably, a number of composers, without prejudice, one may hope, to a lot of others who affect us less deeply. The incredibly rich repertoire made available to all lovers of music, no matter how remote the place in which they live, on long-playing records, virtually throws open the entire world of music: and one's adventures in it are limited only by one's financial resources. But gradually, as I have suggested, we form our preferences, choosing those composers whose works will be 'lamps for my gloom, hands guiding where I stumble': and as we have come to love them so much it seems only natural to want to know not only more about their music but also what manner of men they were, what the surroundings were like in which they worked and lived, what was their historical background, what they looked like, and so forth. And so books about them, that can be trusted to tell the truth, should become a necessity, not a luxury.

Mozart (in this year of his bi-centenary) is a case in point. There have already been available for a number of years two books about him of exceptional interest and value, Eric Blom's volume in the *Master Musicians* series and Alfred Einstein's larger book *Mozart, his life and character*, in an excellent translation from the German. In the first part of Einstein's book, Mozart comes before us as traveller, genius, human being, Catholic and Freemason, while the remainder of the book discusses him as musician and composer. We can complete that vivid picture by turning to the composer's letters which, as Professor Einstein says, are 'the liveliest, least dressed-up, most genuine letters ever written by a musician—we really know Mozart the man'.

A recently published selection of these letters, taken from Emily Anderson's superb three volume edition and edited by Eric Blom, is fortunately now available to everyone in a Penguin book. It is always dangerous to read a man into his music but also foolish to abstract him wholly from it and those lovers of Mozart's music who may have been puzzled by some of the dark places in his work—for example, his G minor Symphony—will surely understand them better when they come across these passages from two letters written in the year before and in the year of his death. 'If people could see into my heart, I should feel almost ashamed. To me everything is cold—cold as ice': and, 'I can't describe what I have been feeling—a kind of emptiness, which hurts me dreadfully—a kind of longing, which is never satisfied, which never ceases, and which persists, nay, rather increases daily . . .'

That is one aspect of Mozart: there emerge also his gaiety, his touching and constant love for his wife, his opinions on the problems of operatic composition, and a wealth of other things that illuminate his character, art, and time.

Mozart is, no doubt, an exceptional case—though both Beethoven's and Wagner's letters make fascinating reading —but even in the case of composers not given to letter writing and whose exterior circumstances were humdrum, a worth-while biography can be enormously rewarding and inspiring. Albert Schweitzer's book on J. S. Bach is a case in point, and I well remember the mounting excitement with which I read it in my student days and with what quickened interest and affection it sent me back to the composer's music.

Composers are not given to writing autobiographies— Wagner, Berlioz, and Stravinsky are among the notable exceptions—but there are many performers, especially singers, who have done so, with results that vary from naive records of 'triumphant tours' to the genuinely informing and revealing.

The lists that follow will show how well music lovers are catered for in the matter of histories of music, and of books, analytical and descriptive, about different categories of music, with Donald Tovey's six volumes of *Essays in Musical Analyses* as a shining example of how to deal with this most difficult subject.

Some sort of musical dictionary should be on the shelves

of every music lover, and here too there is an ample choice. Learned judges in court may ask 'what is sul ponticello'? We, at home, should have no need to do so!

If, as William Blake thought, music, painting and poetry are 'Man's ways of conversing with Paradise' then to be well read about the art to which we particularly incline will surely enable us to take a more intelligent part in those conversations than might otherwise be the case. And that is what books on music are for.

In compiling the reading list the difficulty has been, of course, not what to put in but what to leave out: and there is, it must therefore be remembered, a number of books of merit that could not, for reasons of space be included. It has also not been easy to be consistent in the listing of books according to their category where that category is not well defined, but it is to be hoped the reader will find his way about without too much labour.

Books that deal mainly with the technics of composing, performing, interpretation, and so forth have, except in one or two cases, been omitted, nor must the reader expect to find in the list reference to such impressive volumes as Gustave Reese's *Music in the Middle Ages* and *Music in the Renaissance*, Alfred Einstein's *The Italian Madrigal*, Robbins Landon's *Haydn*, or *The New Oxford History of Music*.

Some of the books are at present out of print but all of them should be found in any well equipped library, while bargains can often be picked up in secondhand book-shops.

READING LIST

All publishers are London firms except where otherwise stated. So far as possible dates of the latest editions are given. Prices (net and subject to alteration) are those prevailing in March, 1956, and are given only where a book is known to be available new as this list goes to press.

DICTIONARIES OF MUSIC

GROVE'S DICTIONARY OF MUSIC AND MUSICIANS. ed. Eric Blom. 5th edn. 9 vols. Macmillan, 1954. £36 (cloth), £50 (leather).

This standard English work is expanded now from five to nine volumes and thoroughly—if not always sufficiently—revised and reset in new type. A particularly valuable feature of the revision is the increased number of tabulated catalogues of works. '*Grove*' aims at being encyclopaedic and universal and those who are unable to afford so large a work will at least be able to consult it in any self-respecting public library.

SCHOLES, PERCY. *The Oxford Companion to Music.* 9th edn. O.U.P., 1955. 63*s.*

Dr. Scholes's famous book continues on its royal progress—nine editions in seventeen years—a poor man's *Grove* of great value, accurate and eminently readable and sometimes highly entertaining. The new edition has been completely revised and reset, with many additions to text and illustrations.

SCHOLES, PERCY. *The Concise Oxford Dictionary of Music.* O.U.P., 1952. 18*s.*

BLOM, ERIC. *Everyman's Dictionary of Music.* Rev. edn. Dent, 1954. 17*s. 6d.*

Two smaller books priced in everybody's reach. The Scholes volume is the larger of the two and has, in addition, some pictorial and musical illustrations and diagrams.

APEL, WILLIAM. *Harvard Dictionary of Music.* Routledge, 1951. 42*s.*

Long-playing records have stimulated a growing interest in music of the pre-Bach eras and this dictionary, which contains no biographical material, gives an exceptional amount of space to clear definitions of technical terms met with in the music of earlier times.

HISTORY

General

LANG, P. H. *Music in Western Civilisation*. Dent, 1942. 63*s*.

A large volume of over 1000 pages and one of the great books of our time. It has a particular value in relating music to the social and political conditions of its times and to philosophy, literature and the other arts. There is a number of illustrations but no musical examples.

EINSTEIN, A. *A Short History of Music*. Cassell, 1948. 8*s*. 6*d*.; with music examples, 14*s*.; illustrated edition, 1953. 30*s*.

The illustrated edition has over 200 pictures but no musical examples.

SACHS, C. *A Short History of World Music*. Dobson, 2nd edn., 1952. New edition in preparation.

A useful volume which will presumably have sundry previous inaccuracies remedied in its forthcoming new edition.

SCHOLES, PERCY. *The Listener's History of Music*. 3 vols. O.U.P., 1943–50. 25*s*. the set.

These admirable volumes, which are illustrated with pictures and musical examples and cost only a few shillings each, are designed for 'any concert-goer, gramophonist or radio listener' and provide the best popular history of music to be had.

Particular (excluding works of a highly specialised character and those to be found in series).

WALKER, E. *A History of Music in England*. 3rd edn. O.U.P., 1952. 40*s*.

ABRAHAM, G. *A Hundred Years of Music*. 2nd edn. Duckworth, 1949. 21*s*.

Professor Abraham describes this very readable volume as 'The Triumph, Decline and Fall of Musical Romanticism'. It covers the span from 1830 to 1936.

12

COOPER, M. *French Music*. O.U.P., 1951. 25s.

From the death of Berlioz to the death of Fauré, a period about which little has been written in detail.

DEMUTH, N. *Musical Trends in the Twentieth Century*. Rockliff, 1952. 35s.

A useful study of 'certain composers who may justly be said to have played a part in the history of world music' since the beginning of this century. It contains portraits and musical illustrations.

OPERA

STREATFIELD, R. A. *The Opera*. 6th rev. edn. Routledge, 1948. 12s. 6d.

First published in 1905 and brought up to date by E. J. Dent in 1948, this book—a sketch of the development of opera with descriptions of all works in the modern repertory and many others—retains its value as a readable and reliable guide.

DENT, E. J. *Opera*. Rev. edn. Penguin (Pelican), 1949. 2s. 6d.

Rightly described as a stimulating guide to the nature and development of opera, and amusingly illustrated.

ORCHESTRA

CARSE, A. VON A. *The Orchestra in the Eighteenth Century*. Heffer, 1940. 10s. 6d.

An illuminating essay on the formation and development of the orchestra, its repute, personnel, status, direction, etc., in the eighteenth century. It makes one listen to the orchestral works of Bach and his sons, Haydn and Mozart, with new interest.

—— *The Orchestra from Beethoven to Berloiz*. Heffer, 1948. 30s.

An equally illuminating volume.

HOWES, F. *Full Orchestra*. New edn. Secker & Warburg, 1950. 3s. 6d.

An excellent short introduction to the history of the evolution of the orchestra and its kinds of music.

ULRICH, H. *Symphonic Music*. O.U.P., 1952. 34s.

A concise and well planned survey of symphonic music, of all

13

categories, from the Renaissance to the present. Musical illustrations.

CHAMBER MUSIC

ULRICH, H. *Chamber Music*. O.U.P., 1948. 48s.

This book, uniform with *Symphonic Music*, noted above, is sub-titled 'the growth and practice of an intimate art' and usefully surveys chamber music from 1600 to the present.

SONGS

MOORE, G. *Singer and Accompanist*. Methuen, 1953. 25s.

Notes, with copious musical illustrations, on the performance of fifty songs by English, French, German, Spanish, Norwegian and Russian composers. A book full of wisdom and artistic insight, the fruit of immense experience.

GREENE, H. PLUNKET. *Interpretation in Song*. Macmillan, 1912. 15s.

A book no singer should be without and one to interest all lovers of song.

PIANO

DALE, K. *Nineteenth-Century Piano Music*. O.U.P., 1954. 25s.
Musical illustrations.

HUTCHESON, E. *The Literature of the Piano*. Hutchinson, 1950.

A valuable guide for amateur and student on the literature of the piano from before Bach to the present day. Musical illustrations.

JAZZ

HARRIS, REX. *Jazz*. Penguin (Pelican), 1952. 2s. 6d.

HOBSON, W. *American Jazz Music*. Dent, 1940.

GRAMOPHONE RECORDS

SACKVILLE-WEST, E., and SHAWE-TAYLOR, D. *The Record Guide*. Rev. edn. Collins, 1955. 35s.

An invaluable guide to the available repertory of gramophone records. A supplemental volume (12s. 6d.) includes all the more important issues up to mid-1955.

CHURCH MUSIC

FELLOWES, EDMUND. *English Cathedral Music*. Methuen, 4th edn., 1949. 18s.

From Edward VI to Edward VII.

ENGLISH MADRIGALS

FELLOWES, EDMUND. *The English Madrigal Composers*. 2nd edn. O.U.P., 1948. 30s.

Indispensable books for students of these subjects.

ANALYTICAL GUIDES

TOVEY, Sir DONALD. *Essays in Musical Analysis*. 6 vols. O.U.P., 1935–39. Each 18s.

—— *Essays in Musical Analysis: Chamber Music*. O.U.P., 1944. 18s.

—— *Musical Articles from the Encyclopaedia Britannica*. O.U.P., 1944. 18s.

The six consecutive volumes of the *Essays* deal with Symphonies (2), Concertos, Illustrative Music, Vocal Music, Supplementary Essays (mainly about orchestral works) with glossary and index to the set. A further volume of essays on *Chamber Music* was issued after Tovey's death and edited by Hubert Foss, who was also responsible for collecting, in yet another volume, all the articles Tovey wrote for the *Encyclopaedia Britannica*. The *Essays* are based on the magnificent programme notes that Tovey wrote for the concert room, informative, profound, witty, sometimes provocative or occasionally (as some may think) wrong-headed, but at all times immensely stimulating and a musical education in themselves. There are plentiful musical examples.

NEWMARCH, R. *The Concert Goer's Library of Descriptive Notes*. O.U.P., 6 vols. 1928–48. Each 6s.

Six small volumes of programme notes witten for the Henry Wood Promenade Concerts, straightforward accounts, somewhat old-fashioned, but serviceable. No musical illustrations.

HILL, RALPH. ed. *The Concerto*. Penguin (Pelican), 1955. 3*s*. 6*d*.

—— *The Symphony*. Penguin (Pelican), 1955. 3*s*. 6*d*.

ROBERTSON, ALEC. ed. *Chamber Music*. Penguin (Pelican), forthcoming.

Three Pelican volumes, covering in each case the general repertoire. Many musical examples.

NEWMAN, E. *Wagner Nights*. Putnam, 1949. 35*s*.

—— *Opera Nights*. Putnam, 1943. 25*s*.

—— *More Opera Nights*. Putnam, 1954. 42*s*.

The two volumes of *Opera Nights* are devoted to repertoire works ranging from Gluck's *Orfeo* to Berg's *Wozzeck* and some operas very rarely performed to-day, such as Meyerbeer's *Les Huguenots* and Berlioz's *Les Troyens*. Each opera, as also in the Wagner volume, is preceded by an essay on its origins, these essays being at once immensely erudite and most readable. There are many pictorial and musical illustrations.

KOBBÉ, G. *Complete Opera Book*. Rev. edn. Putnam, 1954. 45*s*.

A new edition of this well-known book, edited and revised by the Earl of Harewood, who has added a number of analyses by himself on works omitted by, or unknown to, the original author and later editors. The portraits in the old edition are replaced by new ones of singers of our time.

SALTER, L. *Going to the Opera*. Phoenix House, 1955. 9*s*. 6*d*.

WILLIAMS, S. *Come to the Opera*. Hutchinson, 1948. 12*s*. 6*d*.

—— *In the Opera House*. Hutchinson, 1952. 16*s*.

Three popular books on the standard repertoire operas and, in Lionel Salter's book, on what goes on behind and in front of the footlights in the opera house.

COMPOSERS

Series

The list below gives the generic titles of series of volumes, small and large, dealing with composers and their works, with mention of some outstanding volumes. It must be left to the reader to discover, from the lists printed on the covers of the books in question, the full range of composers covered.

MASTER MUSICIANS, ed. Eric Blom. Dent. Each 10s. 6d.
These inexpensive books are wonderful value. Each of them
contains, besides accounts of the life and of the whole output
of the composer concerned, four appendices, a calendar, a
catalogue of works, personalia, and a bibliography. There are
many musical illustrations. Some of the outstanding volumes
among the twenty-five so far issued are *Beethoven*: Marion
Scott; *Bizet*: Winton Dean; *Chopin*: Arthur Hedley; *Haydn:*
Rosemary Hughes; *Mozart*: Eric Blom; *Purcell:* J. A. Westrup;
and *Verdi:* Dyneley Hussey.

THE MUSIC MASTERS, ed. A. L. Bacharach; Vol. I. *Sixteenth
Century to the Time of Beethoven.* Cassell (Fridberg) 1948. 18s.
Vol. 2. *After Beethoven to Wagner.* Cassell, 1951. 21s. Vol. 3.
Borodin to Mascagni. Cassell, 1952, 25s. Vol. 4. *Richard Strauss
to Benjamin Britten.* Cassell, 1954. 25s.
The four large volumes of this series, each about 300 pages and
mainly biographical, cover a very wide range of composers and
include such names as Cornelius, Gade and Spohr, in addition
to all the more familiar ones. There are no musical examples.

THE HERITAGE OF MUSIC, ed. Hubert J. Foss. O.U.P., 3 vols.
1925–51. Each 12s. 6d.
In the three volumes of this series the emphasis is laid on the
music rather than on the life of the composer and most of the
essays, by well-known writers, are of a distinguished character.
Thus we have Terry's essay on Palestrina (Vol. 1), Tovey's on
Gluck (Vol. 2) and Dent's on Rossini (Vol. 3) which alone are
worth the price of each book. There is a small number of
musical examples.

SYMPOSIUM, ed. Gerald Abraham. O.U.P., 5 vols. 1952–54. Each
18s.
This series of, at present, five volumes, is planned on much the
same lines as Dent's *Master Musicians*, except that biography
is replaced by an essay on the man and that the treatment of the
works is more detailed. Composers represented are: *Handel,
Grieg, Schubert, Schumann, Sibelius, Tchaikovsky.*

General

LEONARD, R. A. *The Stream of Music.* Jarrolds (Norwich), 1945.
18s.
A useful book which traces the development of the art of music

during the past three hundred years by basing it on the lives, personalities and works of most of the great composers from Bach to Stravinsky.

FRANK, ALAN. *Modern British Composers.* Dobson, 1953. 7s. 6d.
Excellent short essays on our modern school of composers.

HUSSEY, DYNELEY. *Some Composers of Opera.* O.U.P., 1955. 7s. 6d.
Short essays on composers of opera from Monteverdi to Puccini and including Donizetti, Bellini and Gounod.

SHORE, BERNARD. *Sixteen Symphonies.* Longmans, 1949. 21s.
Haydn to Walton. A first-rate book. Pictorial and musical illustrations.

CARDUS, NEVILLE. *Ten Composers.* Cape, 1945. 10s. 6d.
Schubert to Sibelius. Very readable.

GRAY, CECIL. *A Survey of Contemporary Music.* O.U.P., 1928.
From Strauss to Bartók and Schoenberg. Very provocative and stimulating.

Johann Sebastian Bach

TERRY, C. S. *Bach.* 2nd edn. O.U.P., 1933. 35s.
The standard work in the English language and a mine of information. There are 76 fine photographs of persons, places and things.

PARRY, C. H. *Johann Sebastian Bach.* Rev. edn., Putnam. 1927. 15s.
A condensed life, but a comprehensive and admirable discussion of the works, with pictorial and musical illustrations.

SCHWEITZER, A. *J. S. Bach.* 2 vols. 8th edn., Black, 1952. 50s.
Translated from the German by Ernest Newman.
A classic which subsequent criticism has not robbed of its illuminating and inspiring character. Bach's works and their background and performance are discussed in full. The life itself is briefly treated. There is a large number of musical examples.

DICKENSON, A. E. F. *The Art of Bach*. Duckworth, 1936.

A useful small guide to the music.

Bela Bartók

STEVENS, H. *Life and Music of Bela Bartók*. O.U.P., 1953. 45*s*.

With illustrations and musical examples. An excellent book on this great composer.

Johannes Brahms

GEIRINGER, K. *Brahms*. Allen & Unwin, 2nd edn., 1948. 21*s*.

A fine study of Brahms as man and musician, with pictorial and musical illustrations.

Ludwig van Beethoven

BEKKER, P. *Beethoven*. Dent, 1925.

RIEZLER, W. *Beethoven*. Forrester, 1938.

Other than Marion Scott's small volume in the *Master Musicians* series, the two books mentioned above (both translations from the German) are the best available, on a larger scale, dealing with life and works. There are no musical examples in Bekker's volume.

GROVE, G. *Beethoven, Schubert, Mendelssohn*. Macmillan, 1951. 25*s*.

Grove's famous articles, taken from his equally famous *Dictionary of Music and Musicians* (they are replaced by new contributions in the 1954 edition), reprinted with a preface by Eric Blom.

—— *Beethoven and his Nine Symphonies*. Novello, 1896. 21*s*.

HAMBURGER, M., ed. *A Selection of Beethoven's Letters, Journals and Conversations*. Thames & Hudson, 1951. 21*s*.

Hector Berlioz

WOTTON, T. *Hector Berlioz*. O.U.P., 1935.

William Byrd

FELLOWES, E. H. *William Byrd*. 2nd edn. O.U.P., 1948. 25*s*.

A book about the life and works of one of our greatest composers by an author who did splendid pioneer work for Tudor music.

Benjamin Britten

WHITE, E. W. *Benjamin Britten.* Boosey & Hawkes, 1954. 14*s.*

MITCHELL, D., and KELLER, H. *Benjamin Britten.* Rockcliff, 1954. New edition in preparation.

The first of these books is a short sketch of the composer's life and work; the second, to which both editors, as well as other authors, contribute, is a full-length—and sometimes over adulatory—study. Both books are illustrated and contain musical examples.

Frederic Chopin

CORTOT, A. D. *In Search of Chopin.* Nevill, 1951. 15*s.*

A slight book, but of special interest as coming from a great interpreter of Chopin.

WIERZYNSKI, K. *The Life and Death of Chopin.* Cassell, 1951. 21*s.*

A biography by one of Poland's great poets, without any romantic nonsense in it.

François Couperin

MELLERS, W. *François Couperin and the French Classical Tradition.* Dobson, 1950. 30*s.*

The first book on Couperin in the English language and one that will not easily be surpassed. Life and works are fully discussed. Musical examples.

Claude Debussy

MYERS, R. H. *Debussy.* Duckworth, 1948. 6*s.*

One of the *Great Lives* series, with an account also of the music.

Frederick Delius

FENBY, E. *Delius as I knew him.* Bell, 1936.

HUTCHINGS, A. F. *Delius.* Macmillan, 1948. 12*s.* 6*d.*

WARLOCK, P. *Frederick Delius.* New edn., Bodley Head, 1952. 15*s.*

The new edition of Peter Warlock's book has additions and comments by Hubert Foss. The music is more fully discussed in the volume by Professor Hutchings, and Eric Fenby provides a deeply interesting account of the time he spent as the composer's amanuensis.

Edward Elgar

MAINE, B. *Elgar, his Life and Works*. 2 vols. Bell, 1933.

McVEAGH, D. *Edward Elgar*. Dent, 1955. 18s.

YOUNG, P. *Elgar, O. M.* Collins, 1955. 30s.
Basil Maine devotes one volume to the life and one to the works. Percy Young has had special access to letters and diaries, manuscripts and unpublished pieces. Miss McVeagh's much shorter book is exceptionally good on the music.

Manuel de Falla

PAHISSA, J. *Manuel de Falla*. Museum Press, 1954. 15s.
An admirable account of the composer and his music by one of his countrymen.

César Franck

VALLAS, L. *César Franck*. Harrap, 1951. 15s.
A revealing portrait which differs much from the stained glass figure in D'Indy's biography.

George Frederic Handel

DENT, E. J. *Handel*. Duckworth, 1934. 6s.

FLOWER, N. *George Frederic Handel*. Cassell, 1947. 27s. 6d.

WEINSTOCK, H. *Handel*. Knopf (U.S.A.), 1946.
The first two books are biographical, Professor Dent's being one of the series of Duckworth's *Great Lives*. Weinstock's book, which has pictorial but no musical illustrations, includes a considerable amount of comment on the music.

YOUNG, P. *The Oratorios of Handel*. Dobson, 1949. 18s.
Many musical examples.

Joseph Haydn

GEIRINGER, K. *Haydn, a Creative Life in Music*. Allen & Unwin, 1947. 21s.

JACOB, H. E. *Joseph Haydn, his Art, Times and Glory*. Gollancz. 1950.

Geiringer's book is on a level with Einstein's *Mozart*: Jacob's is a charming but much less profound volume.

Gustav Holst

HOLST, I. *The Music of Gustav Holst*. O.U.P., 1951. 18*s*.

A very candid account of the composer and his music by his daughter.

Franz Liszt

SEARLE, H. *The Music of Liszt*. Williams & Norgate, 1954. 25*s*.

SITWELL, S. *Liszt*. New edn. Cassell, 1955. 30*s*.

A new edition of Sitwell's fascinating Life.

HUGO, H. E. *The Letters of Liszt to Marie zu Sagn-Wittgenstein*. O.U.P., 1953. 52*s*.

Claudio Monteverdi

REDLICH, H. *Monteverdi*. O.U.P., 1952. 25*s*.

A study of the life and works by an author who has done much to encourage the revival of Monteverdi's music. Pictorial and musical illustrations.

Wolfgang Amadeus Mozart

EINSTEIN, A. *Mozart, his Character and Work*. Cassell, 1956. 25*s*.

MITCHELL, D. *Mozart*. Duckworth, 1934. 6*s*.

HUSSEY, DYNELEY. *Wolfgang Amade Mozart*. Kegan Paul, 1928.

Einstein penetrates deeply into the heart of Mozart's character and work and this fine book should be read by all serious lovers of his music.

BLOM, ERIC, ed. *Mozart's Letters*. Penguin, 1956. 3*s*. 6*d*.

KENYON, MAX, ed. *The Letters of Mozart. A Selection*. Barker, 1956. 16*s*.

SAINT-FOIX, G. DE. *The Symphonies of Mozart*. Dobson, 1947. 8*s*. 6*d*.

GIRDLESTONE, C. M. *Mozart's Piano Concertos*. Cassell, 1948. 25s.

HUTCHINGS, A. *A Companion to Mozart's Concertos*. 2nd edn. O.U.P., 1950. 21s.

Girdlestone's book is a standard work, treating the concertos and their background very fully: Hutchings's volume is not so exhaustive and more adapted to the ordinary music lover.

Carl Nielsen

SIMPSON A. *Carl Nielsen*. Dent, 1952. 21s.

Mainly about Nielsen the symphonist but covering all categories of his music.

Giacomo Puccini

MAREK, G. *Puccini*. Cassell, 1952. 21s.

SPECHT, R. *Puccini*. Dent, 1933.

Marek's book is mainly biographical: Specht deals with the music as well as with the life of the composer. A new book on the music is in preparation by Mosco Carner.

Sergei Rachmaninov

CULSHAW, J. *Rachmaninov*. Dobson, 1949. 10s. 6d.

Maurice Ravel

MANUEL, R. *Ravel*. Dobson, 1947. 10s. 6d.

Two volumes in a series devoted to contemporary composers, the first of which alone has musical examples.

Gioacchino Rossini

TOYE, F. *Rossini*, Barker, 1955. 16s.

Mr. Toye calls his excellent book 'a study in tragic comedy'.

Domenico Scarlatti

KIRKPATRICK, R. *Domenico Scarlatti*. O.U.P., 1953. 63s.

An outstanding book by one of the finest harpsichord players of our time. It contains Kirkpatrick's re-numbering of the sonatas and many pictorial and musical illustrations.

Arnold Schoenberg

LEIBOWITZ, R. *Schoenberg and his School.* Philosophical Library (U.S.A.), 1949.

A useful study of 'the contemporary stage of the language of music' for those interested in the music of Schoenberg, Berg and Webern.

Franz Schubert

EINSTEIN, A. *Schubert.* New edn. Cassell, 1951. 25*s.*

A brief biography and a full treatment of the music with a few musical examples. As illuminating as the same author's book on Mozart.

Jean Sibelius

EKMAN, KARL, *Jean Sibelius.* Wilmer, 1937.

The standard biography.

GRAY, CECIL, *Sibelius*, O.U.P., 1935. 3*s.* 6*d.*

A brief introduction to the man and his music.

See also under BIOGRAPHIES, p. 26.

Johann Strauss

JACOB, H. E. *Johann Strauss, A Century of Light Music.* Rev. edn. Hutchinson, 1949. 18*s.*

Igor Stravinsky

WHITE, E. W. *Stravinsky.* Lehmann, 1947.
The best available critical survey of Stravinsky and his music. Pictorial illustrations.

Pete Ilyitch Tchaikovsky

WEINSTOCK, H. *Tchaikovsky.* Cassell, 1946. 21*s.*
Uniform with the same author's book on Handel and including the results of recent Soviet research.

Ralph Vaughan Williams

FOSS, H. *Ralph Vaughan Williams.* Harrap, 1950. 12*s.* 6*d.*

HOWES, F. *The Music of Ralph Vaughan Williams.* O.U.P., 1954. 25*s.*

YOUNG, P. *Vaughan Williams.* Dobson, 1953. 18s.
Foss's book includes a charming chapter of autobiography by the composer. Howes gives a detailed analytical guide to the works.

Giuseppe Verdi

TOYE, F. *The Life and Works of Verdi.* Heinemann, 1931.
A standard book.

GATTI, C. *Verdi: the Man and his Music.* Gollancz, 1955, 21s.
An excellent portrait of the man but an indifferent account of the music.

Richard Wagner

HADOW, H. *Richard Wagner*, O.U.P. (Home University Library), 1934.

NEWMAN, E. *Life of Wagner.* 4 vols. Cassell, 1933. Vols. 3 & 4 only available at 30s. each.

—— *Wagner as Man and Artist.* Bodley Head, 1920.
Much more information about Wagner the man has appeared since Newman wrote this book and is incorporated into the great *Life:* but the two long chapters on Wagner the composer, in theory and practice, retain their full value.

Hugo Wolf

WALKER, F. *Hugo Wolf.* Dent, 1937. 36s.
A biography, with a full account of the music, of outstanding importance.

AUTOBIOGRAPHIES

BEECHAM, SIR THOMAS. *A Mingled Chime.* New edn. Hutchinson, 1952, 18s.
Leaves from an autobiography, up to 1923, penetrating and witty and leaving one eager for the next instalment.

BERLIOZ, H. *Memoirs of Hector Berlioz.* Dent.
This celebrated book is published in Everyman's Library. A new translation, revised and annotated by Ernest Newman, was published in New York in 1935 and should be issued here.

BUSCH, F. *Pages from a Musician's Life*. Hogarth Press, 1953.

COATES, E. *Sonata in Four Movements*. Heinemann, 1953. 16s.
An autobiography of a happy man.

DE LARA, A. *Finale*. Burke, 1955. 18s.
The special interest of this book, apart from the author's lively personality, lies in the fact that she was a pupil of Clara Schumann and met all the famous musicians of her day.

GERHARDT, E. *Recital*. Methuen, 1953. 18s.
A charming account of the great Lieder singer's career, with a preface by Dame Myra Hess and illustrations.

LEHMANN, LILLI. *On Wings of Song*. Routledge n.d.
An endearing book.

SHORE, B. *The Orchestra Speaks*. Longmans, 1938. 10s. 6d.
The author's experiences, as leader of the violas in the B.B.C. Symphony Orchestra, under a number of eminent conductors.

STRAVINSKY, IGOR. *Chronicle of my Life*. Gollancz, 1936.
The author calls his book 'a true picture of myself' and talks about his music and himself with complete frankness. It goes up to 1935.

SZIGETI, J. *With Strings Attached*. Cassell, 1949. 15s.
Personal experiences in concert life, recording and broadcasting; discussions of violin playing, violinists, composers, etc.

WOOD, SIR HENRY. *My Life of Music*. Gollancz, 1938. 6s.

BIOGRAPHIES

Ferruccio Busoni

DENT, E. J. *Ferruccio Busoni*. O.U.P., 1933.
This deeply interesting biography of a remarkable man and pianist contains a list of his repertoire and a catalogue of his compositions. With it should be read Ferrucio Busoni's *Letters to his Wife*, translated by Rosamund Ley (Edward Arnold, 1938).

Pablo Casals

CORREDOR, J. MA. *Conversations with Casals*. Hutchinson, 1956.
   J. Ma Corredor, compiler of this book, uses the method of the leading question and draws from Casals, one of the greatest living men, his opinions on a great variety of subjects including Bach and the playing of Bach, music of yesterday and today, Casals' reasons for his self-imposed exile, memories of his childhood and so forth.

Enrico Caruso

CARUSO, D. *Enrico Caruso*. Werner Laurie, 1948. 21s.
   An account of his life and death by the great singer's wife.

Kathleen Ferrier

CARDUS, NEVILLE, ed. *Kathleen Ferrier: A Memoir*. Hamish Hamilton, 1954. 12s. 6d.

FERRIER, W. *The Life of Kathleen Ferrier*. Hamish Hamilton, 1955. 15s.
   Winifred Ferrier's life of her famous and greatly loved sister fills in the blank spaces of the *Memoir* to which six of her friends and colleagues contributed (Cardus, Barbirolli, Britten, Henderson, Moore, Walter) and includes a number of her letters and a list of her repertoire.

William Furtwängler

RIESS, C. *William Furtwängler*. Muller, 1955. 15s.
   Poor on the musical side but an interesting portrait of the great conductor.

Fritz Kreisler

LOCHNER, L. P. *Fritz Kreisler*. Rockliff, 1951. 27s. 6d.
   Chatty and well illustrated.

Gustav Mahler

WALTER, BRUNO. *Gustav Mahler*. Kegan Paul, 1936.
   Recollections of Mahler and reflections on his music and work as a conductor by one of his closest friends and colleagues.

MAHLER, ALMA. *Gustav Mahler*, Murray, 1946.

Memories by Mahler's wife together with a number of her husband's letters.

Jean Sibelius

DE TORNE, BENGT. *Sibelius: a close-up*. 1937.

The author was for a time a pupil of Sibelius and has much of interest to say about his teacher in these recollections and anecdotes.

Sir Arthur Sullivan

PEARSON, HESKETH. *Gilbert and Sullivan*. Penguin Books.

SULLIVAN, H., and FLOWER, N. *Sir Arthur Sullivan: His Life, Letters and Diaries*. New edn. Cassell, 1950, 12s. 6d.

Sir Richard Terry

ANDREWS, HILDA. *Westminster Retrospect*. O.U.P., 1948.

A memoir of Sir Richard Terry and of the great work he did at Westminster Cathedral.

Arturo Toscanini

TAUBMAN, H. H. *Arturo Toscanini*. Odhams, 1951. 15s.

A full-length and illuminating portrait.

Sir Donald Francis Tovey

GRIERSON, MARY. *Donald Francis Tovey*. O.U.P., 1952. 21s; paper covers, 10s. 6d.

A biography based on letters, and occasionally a disturbing one.

Sir Henry Wood

WOOD, JESSIE. *The Last Years of Henry J. Wood*. Gollancz, 1954. 12s. 6d.

ESSAYS

COLLES, H. C. *Essays and Lectures*. O.U.P., 1945.

FURTWÄNGLER, W. *Concerning Music*. Boosey & Hawkes, 1953. 8s. 6d.

HAMLICK, E. *Vienna's Golden Years of Music*. Gollancz, 1951.

An extremely interesting selection of reviews and essays, made by Harry Pleasants, of a critic too often dismissed as Wagner's chief adversary. Bach, Brahms, Liszt, Humperdinck, Richard Strauss and Verdi, and of course Wagner, are among the composers whose works are noticed.

SCHOENBERG, A. *Style and Idea*. Williams & Norgate.

SHAW, G. BERNARD. *Music in London*, 1890–94. 3 vols. Constable, 1932. Each 15s.

· *London Music in* 1888–89. Constable, 1937.

Although the names of many of the artists and many of the works mentioned may be unknown, even by repute, to the reader these sparkling, witty and sometimes profound criticisms will prove an enduring delight.

STRAUSS, R. *Recollections; Reflections*. Boosey & Hawkes. 1953. 8s. 6d.

TOVEY, SIR DONALD. *Essays and Lectures on Music*. O.U.P., 1949.

VAUGHAN WILLIAMS, A. *Some Thoughts on Beethoven's Choral Symphony, etc.* O.U.P., 1953. 15s.

This list could be much enlarged. There is rewarding reading in all these books.

INDEX OF AUTHORS

30

31

For EU product safety concerns, contact us at Calle de José Abascal, 56–1°,
28003 Madrid, Spain or eugpsr@cambridge.org.

www.ingramcontent.com/pod-product-compliance
Ingram Content Group UK Ltd.
Pitfield, Milton Keynes, MK11 3LW, UK
UKHW040944090126
466816UK00019B/281